"博学而笃志，切问而近思。"

（《论语》）

博晓古今，可立一家之说；
学贯中西，或成经国之才。

复旦博学·复旦博学·复旦博学·复旦博学·复旦博学·复旦博学

内容简介

　　《药学概要》(*The Essentials of Pharmacy*)是以学科主题为引领的新医科学科通识英语教材,适合高等医科院校的本科生及相应英语程度的药科专业的学生使用。教材8个章节的学科内容包括药学概述、药物基本知识、药物研发、药物临床应用、药物涉及的法律和伦理问题、药物安全监管、药物研发与应用的未来趋势、药学教育与职业发展等多个方面,并以读写译视听一体化的形式展开教学。

　　以学科概念为核心的结构化教材,把学科专业内容融入医科英语教学中,让医科英语教学融入学生专业知识体系中,满足不同学科专业学生的学习需求并帮助他们实现学习目标,使英语教学促进学科素养得到有效落实。

新医科学通识英语

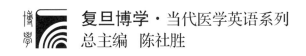

复旦博学·当代医学英语系列
总主编 陈社胜

The Essentials of Pharmacy

药学概要

总主编 陈社胜

主　编 关　庆　金　锋　马芬芬　辛晓明

副主编 谢　倩　张田仓　葛　露　付智茜

编　者（按姓氏笔画排序）

马芬芬 (复旦大学附属浦东医院)

付智茜 (川北医学院)

华　维 (贵州中医药大学)

关　庆 (哈尔滨医科大学大庆校区)

杜　艳 (山西医科大学药学院)

杜　颖 (贵州中医药大学)

杨　芳 (昆明医科大学)

辛晓明 (上海健康医学院)

张田仓 (内蒙古医科大学)

张　莉 (西安医学院)

陈社胜 (复旦大学)

林芳婷 (哈尔滨医科大学大庆校区)

金　锋 (贵州中医药大学)

金　蕾 (昆明医科大学海源学院)

葛　露 (辽宁医药职业学院)

曾熙然 (昆明医科大学海源学院)

谢　倩 (四川卫生康复职业学院)

潘梦妮 (昆明医科大学)

戴玥赟 (山西医科大学)

复旦大学 出版社

序

　　新医科是国家为适应新一轮科技革命和产业变革的要求,提出的从治疗为主到兼具预防、治疗、康养的生命健康全周期的医学发展新理念。2018 年 8 月,中共中央、国务院在关于新时代教育改革发展的重要文件中首次正式提出"新医科"概念。国务院办公厅在 2020 年发布了《关于加快医学教育创新发展的指导意见》,强调"以新医科统领医学教育创新,优化学科专业结构,体现"大健康"理念和新科技革命内涵,对现有专业建设提出理念内容、方法技术、标准评价的新要求,建设一批新的医学相关专业,强力推进医科与多学科深度交叉融合。"为了应对新科技革命的挑战,提高医药卫生服务质量和效率,新医科成为医学教育创新发展的当务之急。

　　医学教育发展新医科的主要目的包括:

　　1. 培养具有创新精神和实践能力的医药卫生人才:新医科强调跨学科、创新型的人才培养模式,旨在培养具备扎实医药卫生基础、广泛人文素养和创新能力的医药卫生人才。

　　2. 推动医学与现代科技的深度融合:新医科鼓励将现代信息技术、人工智能等先进技术应用于医学药卫生领域,以提高医疗服务质量和效率。

　　3. 促进医药卫生事业的可持续发展:新医科关注人口健康、公共卫生等问题,致力于推动医药卫生事业的可持续发展。

　　4. 提升国际竞争力:新医科倡导国际化的教育理念和实践,旨在培养具有国际视野和竞争力的医药卫生人才,提升中国在国际医药卫生领域的话语权和影响力。

　　新医科强调科学、人文、工程的交叉融合,并致力于培养适应人工智能与信息时代医药卫生的复合型人才。药学作为一个分支,在新医科的建设和发展中有其独特的地位和作用。药学作为一门学科,它与医学领域内的其他学科,如预防医学、基础医学、临床医学、康复医学、保健医学等构成了医学这一大的学科门类。作为现代医学科学的一个重要组成部分,药学涵盖了药物的研发、生产、分发、使用和管理等多个方面。药学不仅关注药物的化学结构、药理作用和药效学,还包括药物的安全性、有效性、合理使用以及药物政策和法规。

　　随着医学和科技的发展,药学领域也在不断扩展,包括但不限于临床药学、药物化学、药物分析、药物制剂、药物经济学、药物信息学等子领域。这些领域的发展对于提高医疗服务质量、推动个性化医疗和精准医疗具有重要意义。因此,药学在新医科中占据了不可或缺的地位。

新医科学科通识英语课程的特色之一,是把医药学科的新发展内容注入英语教学中,使英语教学与学科新发展内容学习相融合,学生的学科专业知识学习与英语应用能力提升相融合。以药学学科知识为学习内容的英语教学,对于医科院校药学相关专业的学生有着多方面的意义。

首先,英语是信息的载体,而大量的医药卫生信息和研究成果是以英语为主要语言发布的。如果能把药学知识与技术的学习与英语学习结合起来,学生可以直接阅读和理解这些英语文献资料,及时获取最新的医药技术和研究成果。

其次,药学在医药卫生服务方面起着越来越重要的作用。熟练的英语听说读写能力可以帮助药学专业人员与来自世界各地的同行进行交流和合作。这样不仅可以拓宽视野,学习和借鉴国际上先进的经验和方法,而且还能够加强国际间的医药卫生合作,共同应对全球性的医药卫生问题。

第三,在药物研究和创新方面,掌握药学英语可以跟踪国际最新的医药技术进展,从而及时引进和应用医药新技术,提高我国医药卫生发展水平和医药卫生事业管理成效。

此外,以医药技术知识为学习内容的英语教学,给相关学科的大学生带来的益处可能还包括:更好的就业前景,增进跨文化理解,促进个人成长。

综上所述,随着医药卫生向高度信息化和智能化方向发展,编者们为药学学科编写定制型课程教材,体现了新医科学科通识英语教学"面向学生、面向世界、面向未来"宗旨,服务于国家发展战略、学校办学目标、院系人才培养目标和学生个性化发展的需求。以学科大概念为核心的结构化教材,把学科专业的内容融入医科英语教学中,让医科英语教学融入学生专业知识结构中。这种以学科主题为引领的定制型课程教材,旨在满足特定学习群体的需求并帮助他们实现学习目标,也将促进学科素养的有效落实。

新医科学科通识英语教材《药学概要》是编者们英语教学理念创新的体现,也是编者们对新医科学科通识英语教学理论研究及实践的新成果。

为此,欣然以序祝贺。

复旦博学·当代医学英语系列

总主编 陈社胜

2024 年 3 月

前　言

　　《药学概要》(*The Essentials of Pharmacy*)是创新型新医科学科通识英语教材,适合高等医科院校的本科生及相应英语程度的药科专业的学生使用。

　　国务院办公厅在 2020 年发布了《关于加快医学教育创新发展的指导意见》,强调"以新医科统领医学教育创新,优化学科专业结构,体现'大健康'理念和新科技革命内涵,对现有专业建设提出理念内容、方法技术、标准评价的新要求,建设一批新的医学相关专业,强力推进医科与多学科深度交叉融合。"

　　本教材以教育部关于深化本科教育教学改革全面提高人才培养质量的意见(教高〔2019〕6 号)、教育部关于一流本科课程建设的实施意见(教高〔2019〕8 号)、《健康中国 2030 规划纲要》、2020 年版《大学英语教学指南》等为依据,以"学科专业＋语言学习"相融合的创新体例编写。《药学概要》英语教材的学科内容包括:药学概述、药物基本知识、药物研发、药物临床应用、药物涉及的法律和伦理问题、药物安全监管、药物研发与应用的未来趋势、药学教育与职业发展等 8 大方面。

　　新医科学科通识英语教材的特色之一是学科专业内容教学与医科英语教学相融合;学生学科专业知识学习与英语应用能力提升相融合;并将专业词汇拓展、术语构词学习、英语结构与功能应用、视听能力提升、读写译技能发展等多方面融合一体,使学生学之有味,学之有获,学之有用。

　　《药学概要》教材可用于 45～72 课时教学。教材由教学用书(纸质)、电子版教师参考、互联网音视频资源 3 个部分组成。教学所需影像视听资料、教师教学电子版参考资源等可向复旦大学出版社索取。

　　编者衷心感谢复旦大学出版社在推动新医科英语教育发展创新过程中持续的努力与大力支持,同样感谢新医科英语教材使用者的教学体验及建设性意见,使新医科学科通识英语教材能更完善地应用于大学新医科英语教学中。

编者

2024 年 3 月

CONTENTS

Chapter VI　Safety Regulation of Drugs

Chapter VII　Future Trends in Drug Development and Application

Chapter VIII　Pharmacy Education and Career Development

Appendix

Overall Introduction to Pharmacy

1.1 Overview of the Development of Pharmaceutical Science

The development of **pharmaceutical** science has been a long and **fascinating** journey, **spanning** thousands of years. It has **witnessed** numerous significant events that have shaped the field and contributed to the **advancement** of medicine as we know it today. Here is a brief **overview** of the development history of pharmaceutical science:

1. What contributed to the advancement of pharmaceutical science?

Ancient times (before 2000 BC): The earliest known use of **herbal** medicine dates back to ancient **Egypt**,

2. When was the earliest known use of herbal medicine?

---

pharmaceutical /ˌfɑːrməˈsuːtɪkl/ *adj.*　　制药的;配药的
fascinating /ˈfæsɪneɪtɪŋ/ *adj.*　　极有吸引力的;迷人的
span /spæn/ *v.*　　横跨;跨越;包括
witness /ˈwɪtnəs/ *v.*　　见证;目击
advancement /ədˈvænsmənt/ *n.*　　发展;推动;提升
overview /ˈəʊvərvjuː/ *n.*　　概观;总的看法;回顾
herbal /ˈhɜːbl/ *adj.*　　药草的;草本的
Egypt /ˈɪdʒəpt/ *n.*　　埃及

where **remedies** were **prescribed** for various **ailments** using natural substances found in plants, animals, and minerals. These remedies were often combined and **tailored** according to the patient's needs.

Ancient **Greece** and Rome (2000 BC – 476 AD): During this period, Greek and Roman **physicians** developed a system of medicine based on **observation** and **experimentation**. They discovered many **medicinal properties** of plants, such as the **antipyretic** qualities of **feverfew**, which are still used today in modern medicine.

Middle Ages (476 AD – 1453): During this time, pharmaceutical knowledge was **primarily** passed down orally through word-of-mouth, making it difficult to maintain a **consistent** standard of practice. Medicine also became more specialized, with doctors specializing in surgery, **pharmacology**, and other areas of **expertise**.

3. What system of medicine did ancient Greek and Roman physicians develop?

4. How was pharmaceutical knowledge passed down during the Middle Ages?

---

remedy /ˈremədɪ/ n.		药品;治疗方法
prescribe /prɪˈskraɪb/ v.		开处方;给医嘱;规定
ailment /ˈeɪlmənt/ n.		疾病;病痛;微恙
tailor /ˈteɪlər/ v.		量身打造;按需定制
Greece /griːs/ n.		希腊
physician /fɪˈzɪʃn/ n.		医生;内科医生
observation /ˌɒbzərˈveɪʃn/ n.		观察;观测
experimentation /ɪkˌsperɪmenˈteɪʃn/ n.		实验;试验
medicinal /mɪˈdɪsənəl/ adj.		药用的;治疗的
property /ˈprɒpərtɪ/ n.		特性;属性;财产
antipyretic /ˌæntɪpaɪˈretɪk/ adj.		退热的;退烧的
feverfew /ˈfiːvərfjʊ/ n.		菊科植物;白菊花
primarily /praɪˈmerəlɪ/ adv.		首要地;主要地
consistent /kənˈsɪstənt/ adj.		一致的;连贯的
pharmacology /ˌfɑːməˈkɒlədʒɪ/ n.		药理学;药物学
expertise /ˌekspɜːrˈtiːz/ n.		专长;专门技术;专门知识

Renaissance (1453 – 1700): The **Renaissance** marked a significant turning point in the development of pharmaceutical science. Scientific methods began to be applied to medicine, leading to new discoveries and **innovations**. For example, the work of Andreas Vesalius in the 15th century revolutionized surgery by introducing modern **surgical** techniques and tools.

5. Why is the Renaissance said to remark a significant turning point in the development of pharmaceutical science?

The Age of **Enlightenment** (1700 – 1850): This period saw an **explosion** of scientific knowledge and innovation, particularly in the fields of chemistry and biology. New drugs were **synthesized** from natural **compounds**, paving the way for modern pharmaceuticals. One **notable** discovery was the creation of **quinine** for **malaria** treatment by Alexander Fleming in 1928.

6. In what era did an explosion of scientific knowledge occur?

Industrial Revolution (1850 – 1920): The rise of industry led to significant improvements in drug production, including the development of **standardized** processes for manufacturing drugs and the introduction of chemical **synthesis** for creating new compounds. This era also saw the **emergence** of new **therapeutic**

7. What led to significant improvements of drug production in the period of Industrial Revolution?

Renaissance /ˈreneɪsns/ n.	文艺复兴
innovation /ˌɪnəˈveɪʃn/ n.	创新;新观念;新发明
surgical /ˈsɜːdʒɪkl/ adj.	外科的;外科手术的
Enlightenment /ɪnˈlaɪtnmənt/ n.	启蒙运动;启迪;开导
explosion /ɪkˈspləʊʒn/ n.	激增;突然爆发
synthesize /ˈsɪnθəsaɪz/ v.	合成;人工合成
compound /ˈkɒmpaʊnd/ n.	化合物;混合物
notable /ˈnəʊtəbl/ adj.	值得注意的;显著的
quinine /ˈkwaɪˌnaɪn/ n.	奎宁,金鸡纳霜
malaria /məˈleɪrɪə/ n.	疟疾
standardize /ˈstændərdaɪz/ v.	使标准化;使合乎标准
synthesis /ˈsɪnθəsɪs/ n.	合成;综合
emergence /iˈmɜːrdʒəns/ n.	出现;兴起
therapeutic /ˌθerəˈpjuːtɪk/ adj.	治疗(学)的;疗法的

modalities, such as x-rays and **radiotherapy**.

Second World War (1939 - 1945): In response to the outbreak of war, scientists worked **tirelessly** to develop new drugs for military purposes, including **antibiotics** for **bacterial infections** and blood **plasma transfusions**.

8. Why did scientists work tirelessly to develop new drugs during the Second World War period?

Postwar Era (1945 - present): The **postwar** period saw rapid advances in pharmaceutical science, driven by technological innovations such as mass production techniques, **genetic** engineering, and **biotechnology**. This era has seen the development of **lifesaving** drugs for diseases like cancer, **HIV/AIDS**, and **tuberculosis**, among others.

9. When did pharmaceutical science experience rapid advances?

Throughout its history, pharmaceutical science has continued to evolve and **adapt** to changing circumstances, driven by the **pursuit** of better understanding and the need to improve human health and well-being. Today,

10. What is the driving force for the continued evolution of pharmaceutical science?

---

modality /məʊˈdælətɪ/ *n.*	模式；方式
radiotherapy /ˌreɪdɪəʊˈθerəpɪ/ *n.*	放疗
tirelessly /ˈtaɪələslɪ/ *adv.*	不知疲倦地；坚韧地
antibiotics /ˌæntɪbaɪˈɒtɪks/ *n.*	抗生素，抗菌素
bacterial /bækˈtɪərɪrl/ *adj.*	细菌的；细菌性的
infection /ɪnˈfekʃn/ *n.*	传染；感染；传染病
plasma /ˈplæzmə/ *n.*	血浆；原生质；细胞质
transfusion /trænsˈfjuːʒn/ *n.*	输血
postwar /ˈpəʊstˈwɔː/ *adj.*	战后的
genetic /dʒəˈnetɪk/ *adj.*	遗传的；基因的
biotechnology /ˌbaɪəʊtekˈnɒlədʒɪ/ *n.*	生物技术
lifesaving /ˈlaɪfˌseɪvɪŋ/ *adj.*	救命的；救生的
HIV (Human Immunodeficiency Virus)	艾滋病病毒
AIDS (acquired immune deficiency syndrome)	获得性免疫缺乏综合征(艾滋病)
tuberculosis /tjʊˌbɜːkjəˈləʊsɪs/ *n.*	肺结核；结核病
adapt /əˈdæpt/ *v.*	使适应/适合；改编
pursuit /pərˈsuːt/ *n.*	追求；寻求

pharmaceutical research is focused on developing new treatments for existing diseases while also **addressing** emerging public health challenges such as **infectious** diseases and chronic conditions like **diabetes** and **Alzheimer's disease**.

Language Practice

I. Vocabulary Work

Complete each of the following sentences with a suitable word or expression given below.

fascinating	prescribe	property	innovation
span	ailment	consistent	adapt
witness	observation	surgery	pursuit
overview	medicinal	pharmacology	address
herbal	remedy	expertise	therapeutic

1. The _____ of pharmacology covers the basic principles of drug action, including receptor binding, signal transduction, and physiological response.
2. The _____ administration of medication is crucial for achieving the desired therapeutic effect and avoiding adverse reactions.
3. _____ medication errors and discrepancies is an important aspect of pharmacy practice to ensure patient safety and satisfaction.
4. The clinical trial results were _____ by an independent panel of experts to ensure their validity and reliability.
5. The effectiveness of a medication for a particular _____ is often determined through clinical trials, which involve testing the drug on a group of patients with that condition.

---

address /əˈdres/ v.   解决;处理
diabetes /ˌdaɪəˈbiːtiːz/ n.   糖尿病
Alzheimer's disease /ˈæltshaɪmərz dɪziːz/ n.   阿尔茨海默病

6. The development of new _____ drugs involves a rigorous process of research and testing to ensure their safety and efficacy.

7. In order to maintain their professional competence, pharmacists must continually update their knowledge and _____ through ongoing education and training.

8. One of the key drivers of progress in the field of pharmacy is _____ , as new technologies and techniques are constantly being developed to improve drug discovery and development processes.

9. The shelf life of a medication, or its _____ , refers to the length of time that the drug remains stable and effective for use.

10. Pharmacists must be able to _____ their communication style to effectively convey complex medical information to patients, including instructions on how to take medications safely and effectively.

11. Pharmacists are trained to accurately diagnose and _____ medications based on patients' medical histories, symptoms, and other relevant factors.

12. The development of new drugs often involves identifying novel _____ targets and mechanisms of action.

13. In clinical trials, _____ are made of participants' symptoms and other outcomes in order to evaluate the effectiveness and safety of new drugs.

14. Pharmacists must be knowledgeable about the _____ of medications they dispense, including how they interact with other drugs and substances, in order to provide safe and effective care to their patients.

15. The _____ of new drug discovery is a constant challenge in the field of pharmacy, as researchers seek to identify and develop novel treatments for a wide range of diseases and conditions.

II. Word Building

Study the Prefixes, Suffixes and Roots in the following grid, and then provide the corresponding word based on the given definition.

Prefixes	Meaning		Example
anti-	"against" (反对;对抗)		antibiotics

post-	"after" or "following"（在……后；随后的）	postwar
Suffixes		
-ical	"having the nature or characteristic of"（有……性质或特征）	pharmaceutical
-osis	"a condition or disease"（病情，疾病）	tuberculosis
-ology	"the study of" or "the science of"（……研究，……科学）	pharmacology
Roots		
pharmac	"drug" or "medicine"（药）	pharmacy
bio	"life"（生命）	antibiotics
syn	"together" or "with"（共同，一起）	synthesize

1. a substance that is used to treat bacterial infections by killing or inhibiting the growth of bacteria _____

2. to delay or put off until a later time _____

3. the study of living organisms and their interactions with each other and the environment _____

4. the use of living organisms or biological processes to develop new products or technologies _____

5. the combining of different elements to form a new whole _____

6. a person who prepares and dispenses medicines _____

7. medicines or drugs used for medical purposes _____

8. the study of society, social relationships, and social institutions _____

9. relating to technology or the application of scientific knowledge for practical purposes _____

10. a mental disorder that causes a break with reality _____

III. Structure & Function

An attributive clause（定语从句）is a type of dependent clause that modifies or describes a noun or pronoun in the main clause of a sentence. It usually begins with a relative pronoun such as "who," "whom," "whose," "which," "that," or "where" and provides additional information about the noun or pronoun it modifies. For example：

It has witnessed numerous significant events <u>that have shaped the field and contributed to the advancement of medicine as we know it today</u>.

The earliest known use of herbal medicine dates back to ancient Egypt, <u>where remedies were prescribed for various ailments using natural substances found in plants, animals, and minerals</u>.

They discovered many medicinal properties of plants, such as the antipyretic qualities of feverfew, <u>which are still used today in modern medicine</u>.

Attributive clauses are commonly used in medical literature to provide additional information about a noun or pronoun, and they can achieve several effects.

One effect is to clarify the meaning of a term or concept that may be unfamiliar to readers. For example, an attributive clause can be used to explain what type of drug was used in a study, such as "the antibiotic that was administered intravenously."

Another effect is to provide context for a study or observation. For example, an attributive clause can be used to describe the population being studied, such as "the patients with diabetes who were enrolled in the trial."

Attributive clauses can also be used to indicate the degree or extent of something, such as the severity of a disease or the duration of treatment. For example, an attributive clause can be used to describe the percentage of patients who responded to a treatment with a new drug, such as "the 75% of patients who showed improvement."

Overall, attributive clauses are a useful tool in medical literature because they allow authors to provide more detailed and precise information about their research findings.

Complete the following sentences based on the Chinese given in the brackets, using in each sentences an attributive clause.

1. The researchers are studying _____

    _____ (由当地制药公司的一组科学家开发的新药).

2. The doctor prescribed a new treatment to _____

_____ (其血压对药物没有反应的患者).

3. The clinical trial, _____ (目前正在进行), will test the safety and efficacy of the new drug candidate.

4. The compound _____
_____ (在动物研究中表现出有前景的结果) is being further investigated for its potential therapeutic benefits in humans.

5. The team of experts, _____ (拥有制药开发方面丰富经验), will oversee the project from start to finish.

6. The phase III trial, _____
_____ (患者患有晚期癌症将接受实验性治疗), is set to begin next month.

IV. Audio-visual Exercise

A. Spot Dictation

Listen to a passage twice. Fill in each blank with what you hear while listening.

The history of pharmaceutical science can be traced back to ancient civilizations, where medicinal plants and natural (1) _____ were used for healing purposes. The ancient Egyptians, for example, used herbs such as garlic, honey, and willow bark to treat various (2) _____.

In the Middle Ages, alchemy (炼丹术) played a significant role in pharmaceutical science. Alchemists experimented with various (3) _____ in an attempt to create a universal remedy for all diseases. Some of their discoveries, such as distillation (蒸馏) and the use of chemical (4) _____, laid the foundation for modern pharmacology.

The Renaissance period saw a (5) _____ interest in medicine and pharmacy. Scholars like Paracelsus challenged traditional beliefs about medicine and advocated for a more scientific (6) _____. This led to the development of new drugs and treatments, such as the use of vaccines and (7) _____.

The 19th century marked a significant turning point in pharmaceutical science with the discovery of the (8) _____ of disease. This led to the development of antiseptics and other drugs that could help prevent the (9) _____

_____ . The first synthetic drug, aspirin, was also discovered in this century.

The 20th century saw rapid advancements in pharmaceutical science, with the development of new drug (10) _____ and the introduction of biotechnology. Today, pharmaceutical scientists continue to research new drugs and treatments for (11) _____ of diseases, including cancer, diabetes, and mental health disorders.

Overall, the history of pharmaceutical science has been characterized by (12) _____ , and a constant drive to improve human health and well-being.

B. Visual Comprehension

Watch a video clip three times and decide whether each of the following statements is true（T）or false（F）.

_____ 1. A new drug produces remarkable results against a form of cancer which is usually considered a death sentence.

_____ 2. Former president Jimmy Carter, who was treated for advanced lung cancer with Keytruda, announced later he was cancer-free.

_____ 3. The new drug gives hopes not only to advanced lung cancer patients, but potentially to those suffering melanoma as well.

_____ 4. A new study says 40% of advanced melanoma patients were alive 3 years after taking Keytruda.

_____ 5. Arian Younger Berg is also a living proof of the promise of targeted therapy with Keytruda.

_____ 6. In the U. S. , treatment with Keytruda is very expensive and not covered by insurance.

_____ 7. According to Dr. Stephen Godi, Keytruda is not a cure, although it is an exciting progress.

V. Extended Reading

Read the following dialogue between Dr. Pharmed, a pharmacist, and students about the development of pharmaceutical science, and choose the best answer to each question according to the dialogue.

Dr. Pharmed: Hello, everybody. It's great to have you here. I'm so excited to discuss the development of pharmaceutical science with you today.

Student 1: Hi, Dr. Pharmed. Thank you for inviting us. I'm really interested in this topic. Can you tell us about the history of pharmaceutical science?

Dr. Pharmed: Absolutely! The history of pharmaceutical science dates back to ancient times. In ancient Greece, Egypt and China, people used plants and other natural substances to treat diseases. However, it wasn't until the Middle Ages that drugs began to be prepared and dispensed more systematically.

Student 2: That's fascinating. So what are some of the major milestones in the development of pharmaceutical science?

Dr. Pharmed: One of the most significant milestones was the discovery of penicillin by Alexander Fleming in 1928. Penicillin is an antibiotic that revolutionized the treatment of bacterial infections. It paved the way for the development of other antibiotics and opened up a new era in modern medicine.

Student 3: That's amazing. What are some of the latest advancements in pharmaceutical science?

Dr. Pharmed: In recent years, there have been many exciting advancements in pharmaceutical science. One area of particular interest is precision medicine, which involves the use of targeted drugs and genetic therapies to treat diseases based on their underlying causes.

Student 4: That sounds revolutionary! Are there any future trends or areas of research that are particularly exciting?

Dr. Pharmed: Absolutely! One area that's particularly exciting is the field of nanotechnology. Nanotechnology involves the use of extremely small particles, known as nanoparticles, to deliver drugs to specific parts of the body. This approach has the potential to improve drug delivery and reduce side effects, opening up new possibilities for treatment.

Student 5: That's incredible! Thank you so much for sharing with us today. It's truly eye-opening to learn about the rich history and exciting future of pharmaceutical science.

Dr. Pharmed: Absolutely! I hope this has been a valuable learning experience for you all. Pharmaceutical science is an incredibly dynamic and exciting field, and I'm looking forward to witnessing its continued progress in the future. Thank you for coming and asking questions!

1. According to Dr. Pharmed, the history of pharmaceutical science is traced back to _____ .

   A. ancient Greece

   B. ancient China

   C. ancient Egypt

   D. all of the above

2. Which of the following is NOT a significance of the discovery of penicillin?

   A. It was a natural substance to treat diseases.

   B. It opened up a new era in modern medicine.

   C. It revolutionized the treatment of bacterial infections.

   D. It paved the way for the development of other antibiotics.

3. Precision medicine _____ .

   A. is the latest advancement in pharmaceutical science

   B. relies on the development of pharmaceutical science

   C. involves the use of targeted drugs to treat diseases

   D. has the potential to treat most genetic diseases

4. Which of the following statements is NOT true of nanotechnology?

   A. It is opening up new possibilities for drug research.

   B. It is a revolutionary treatment for genetic diseases.

   C. It has the potential to improve drug delivery.

   D. It has the potential to reduce side effects.

5. Pharmaceutical science _____ .

   A. has a rich history and exciting future

   B. will witness its continued progress

   C. is an incredibly dynamic field

D. is all of the mentioned above

Chapter I   Overall Introduction to Pharmacy   **13**

D. is all of the mentioned above

VI. Topics for Discussion and Essay-writing

1. What do you think is the most exciting advancement in pharmaceutical science?
2. What is the driving force for the continued evolution of pharmaceutical science?
3. What do you think of the pharmaceutical research focus today?

1.2 Overview of the Pharmaceutical Development in China

The history of pharmaceutical development in China can be traced back to ancient times, with a rich tradition of herbal medicine and other natural remedies. Over the centuries, this tradition has been shaped by various cultural, social, and political factors, leading to **significant** advancements in the field of pharmacology.

One of the earliest recorded **events** in Chinese pharmaceutical history is the Shang **Dynasty** (1600 – 1046 BCE), where medicinal plants were used for **healing** purposes. The Huangdi Neijing (*The Yellow Emperor's Inner Canon*), also known as the Canon of **Internal** Medicine, was **compiled** during the Han Dynasty (206 BCE – 220 CE) and is considered one of the most important medical texts in Chinese history. It contains descriptions of various herbs and their therapeutic properties, as well as information on **acupuncture** and other treatments.

During the Tang Dynasty (618 – 907 CE), phar-

1. What tradition is characteristic of the pharmaceutical development in China?

2. Which text is considered one of the most important medical texts in Chinese history?

---

significant /sɪɡˈnɪfɪkənt/ *adj.*   重要的;显著的;意味深长的
event /ɪˈvent/ *n.*   事件;重大事件
dynasty /ˈdaɪnəstɪ/ *n.*   朝代;王朝
healing /ˈhiːlɪŋ/ *n.*   痊愈;愈合;治愈
canon /ˈkænən/ *n.*   精品;真作;规范;原则
The Yellow Emperor's Inner Canon   《黄帝内经》
internal /ɪnˈtɜːrnl/ *adj.*   内部的;体内的;国内的
compile /kəmˈpaɪl/ *v.*   汇编;编制;编纂
acupuncture /ˈækjʊpʌŋktʃər/ *n.*   针刺;针刺疗法

maceutical knowledge continued to expand, and many new medicinal substances were introduced from neighboring countries such as India and **Persia**. The Tang physician Li Shizhen (581 – 682 CE) is considered one of the most **influential figures** in Chinese pharmacology, having **authored** *The Compendium of Materia Medica*, a **comprehensive** guide to medicinal plants and their uses.

3. What is the Compendium of Materia Medica?

In the Song Dynasty (960 – 1279 CE), advances in pharmaceutical technology led to the development of new **manufacturing** techniques, such as the process of **distillation**, which allowed for the production of effective medicines like **camphor** and **musk**. The Song period also saw the establishment of the first **pharmacopoeia**, or official list of **approved** medicinal substances, which helped to standardize the quality and safety of medicines.

4. Who authored this medical text?

5. What advances were made in pharmaceutical technology in the Song Dynasty?

6. When was the first pharmacopoeia established?

The Ming Dynasty (1368 – 1644 CE) and Qing Dynasty (1644 – 1912 CE) witnessed further progress in pharmaceutical research and development, with many

---

Persia /ˈpəːʃə/ *n.*   波斯(现在的伊朗)
influential /ˌɪnfluˈenʃl/ *adj.*   有影响力的;有权势的
figure /ˈfɪɡjər/ *n.*   人物;身影;数字
author /ˈɔːθər/ *v./n.*   创作;撰写;作者
compendium /kəmˈpendɪəm/ *n.*   概要;纲要
The Compendium of Materia Medica   《本草纲目》
comprehensive /ˌkɒmprɪˈhensɪv/ *adj.*   综合性的;全面的
manufacturing /ˌmænjəˈfæktʃərɪŋ/ *n.*   制造;加工;工业
distillation /ˌdɪstɪˈleɪʃn/ *n.*   蒸馏(过程);蒸馏物
camphor /ˈkæmfə/ *n.*   樟脑
musk /mʌsk/ *n.*   麝香
pharmacopoeia /ˌfɑːməkəˈpɪə/ *n.*   药典
approve /əˈpruːv/ *v.*   同意;批准;通过

new drugs being introduced to treat a wide range of diseases. During this time, traditional Chinese medicine (TCM) began to gain **recognition** both **domestically** and internationally, with TCM practitioners traveling **abroad** to share their knowledge and expertise.

In modern times, China has continued to make significant contributions to the field of pharmacology. The founding of the People's Republic of China in 1949 led to the establishment of a national **healthcare** system and the development of new drugs and treatments for various diseases. In recent years, China has become a major player in global pharmaceutical research and development, with many Chinese companies investing heavily in innovative drug discovery and manufacturing technologies.

Notable figures in Chinese pharmaceutical history include Li Shizhen, whose work on traditional Chinese medicine and pharmacology has had a lasting impact on the field; Zhang Zhongjing is known as the "Father of Modern Chinese Medicine" and was a famous traditional Chinese medicine doctor in the early 20th century. He made significant contributions to the development of traditional Chinese medicine, especially in the fields of gynecology and pediatrics; Tu Youyou, who won the Nobel Prize in **Physiology** or Medicine in 2015 for her work on malaria treatment.

7. When did traditional Chinese medicine begin to gain recognition both domestically and internationally?

8. What is evidence of significant contributions China has made in modern times?

9. Who has been mentioned as notable figures in Chinese pharmaceutical history?

---

recognition /ˌrekəɡˈnɪʃn/ *n*.　　　　　认识；识别；认出
domestically /dəˈmestɪklɪ/ *adv*.　　　　在国内；在本国；家庭式
abroad /əˈbrɔːd/ *adv*.　　　　　　　　到国外；在国外
healthcare /ˈhelθkeə/ *n*.　　　　　　　卫生保健
physiology /ˌfɪzɪˈɒlədʒɪ/ *n*.　　　　　生理学；生理（功能）

In conclusion, the history of pharmaceutical development in China is long and complex, **reflecting** the country's rich cultural **heritage** and its **ongoing** contributions to the field of medicine. From ancient herbal remedies to modern drug discovery and development, China has played a **vital** role in shaping the world of pharmacology.

10. What can be concluded about the history of pharmaceutical development in China?

Language Practice

I. Vocabulary Work

Complete each of the following sentences with a suitable word or expression given below.

significant	internal	compendium	approve
event	compile	comprehensive	recognition
healing	acupuncture	distillation	domestically
reflect	influential	figure	healthcare
heritage	vital	physiology	impact

1. Pharmaceutical science has developed a _____ understanding of the molecular mechanisms underlying diseases, leading to the discovery of new drug targets.

2. The approval of a new drug is always an _____ that attracts significant attention from the scientific community and the media.

3. The _____ of scientific literature on the development of new drugs provides a valuable resource for researchers and drug developers.

4. Scientists _____ research findings from multiple sources to gain a

---

reflect /rɪˈflekt/ *v*.　　　　　　反映;表现;反射
heritage /ˈherɪtɪdʒ/ *n*.　　　　　遗产;传统
ongoing /ˈɒngəʊɪŋ/ *adj*.　　　　不间断的;进行的;前进的
vital /ˈvaɪtl/ *adj*.　　　　　　　必要的;至关重要的;充满活力的

comprehensive understanding of a particular disease or therapeutic area.

5. The development of personalized medicine is revolutionizing _____ by providing patients with drugs that are tailored to their specific needs.

6. The clinical trial results _____ a promising trend in the efficacy of the new drug for treating Alzheimer's disease.

7. The discovery of penicillin by Alexander Fleming was a landmark moment in pharmaceutical history and continues to be an _____ example of the power of natural compounds to fight infection.

8. The discovery of a new treatment for a rare disease brought _____ to the researcher who spent years studying the condition.

9. Traditional herbal remedies have played a significant role in the _____ of pharmaceutical development, with many modern drugs based on these ancient treatments.

10. The contributions of _____ like Alexander Fleming to pharmacy are immeasurable, as they paved the way for modern practices in the field.

11. The development of new treatments for rare diseases can have a significant _____ on the quality of life for those affected by these conditions.

12. The regulatory agency will review the safety and efficacy data submitted by the pharmaceutical company before making a decision on whether to _____ the new treatment.

13. Pharmaceutical companies often conduct extensive _____ studies to better understand how a drug affects the body and its various systems.

14. The goal of pharmaceutical development is not only to create new treatments but also to promote _____ and improve patient outcomes.

15. The use of _____ in pharmaceutical development is still relatively new, but there is growing interest in its potential to provide safe and effective alternatives to traditional medications.

II. Word Building

Study the Prefixes, Suffixes and Roots in the following grid, and then provide the corresponding word based on the given definition.

Prefixes	Meaning	Example
ab-	"away from" or "from"（离开；分离）	abroad
manu-	"hand or by hand"（手或用手）	manufacturing
Suffixes		
-ant	"having the qualities of"（有……品质）	significant
-age	"the state or quality of"（名词后缀：状态或性质）	heritage
-ium	"a collection or summary of information"（信息集合或摘要）	compendium
Roots		
signify	"to indicate or mean"（表明；示意）	significant
physio	"related to physiology or physics"（与生理或物理相关的）	physiology
herit	"to receive something from an ancestor"（从祖辈继承）	heritage

1. to refrain from doing something _____

2. something that is passed down from earlier generations _____

3. capable of being inherited _____

4. referring to something that is done by hand _____

5. insufficient quantity or supply; a lack of something needed _____

6. a treatment method that uses physical techniques to help improve or restore movement and function in the body _____

7. able to resist something, such as an infection, a force, or change _____

8. having great importance, meaning, or impact _____

9. to remove or separate from a physical or material form _____

10. a concise collection of information, a condensed overview of a larger work or subject _____

III. Structure & Function

The passive structure widely used in medical literature in English is called the passive voice. The passive voice is used to convey information about the subject of a sentence, rather than the action of the subject. For example：

The history of pharmaceutical development in China <u>has been shaped</u> by various cultural, social, and political factors.

The Canon of Internal Medicine <u>was compiled</u> during the Han Dynasty（206

BCE‐220 CE） *and is considered one of the most important medical texts in Chinese history.*

During the Tang Dynasty（618‐907 CE）, pharmaceutical knowledge continued to expand, and many new medicinal substances were introduced from neighboring countries such as India and Persia.

Scientific methods began to be applied to medicine, leading to new discoveries and innovations.

Over the centuries, this tradition has been shaped by various cultural, social, and political factors.

The passive structure is widely used in medical literature in English for several reasons. One of the main reasons is that the passive voice often provides a more objective and impersonal tone, which is important in scientific writing. By using the passive voice, the focus is shifted from the subject to the action or phenomenon being described, which can help to eliminate subjective biases and emphasize the scientific facts.

Another reason is that the passive structure is often more concise and economical, which is important in technical and medical writing where conciseness and precision are essential. Using the passive voice can eliminate the need to use personal pronouns or specify the subject, making the text easier to read and less cluttered.

Additionally, the passive structure can be used to conceal some messages for stylistic or practical reasons. For example, when writing about experiments or procedures, the passive voice can conceal the identity of the experimenter or provide a more impersonal description of the process.

Overall, the passive structure is widely used in medical literature because it promotes objectivity, conciseness, and concealment of information when necessary.

Translate each of the following sentences into English.

1. 该新药的临床试验由一家知名医疗机构的专业研究团队进行。

2. 报告中使用被动语态是为了强调新药开发研究结果的客观性。

_____

_____

3. 一种新药在投入使用前,必须经过独立的第三方进行安全性和有效性测试。

_____

_____

4. 在撰写科学论文时,采用被动语态是为了保持正式和客观的语气,避免主观意见或偏见。

_____

_____

5. 在决定是否继续进行进一步的测试或上市销售之前,一个专家小组将对临床试验结果进行评估。

_____

_____

IV. Audio-visual Exercise

A. Spot Dictation

Listen to a passage twice. Fill in each blank with what you hear while listening.

The development of pharmaceutical science in China can be traced back to ancient times, where traditional herbal medicines were used for (1) _____ purposes. However, it was not until the 20th century that modern pharmaceutical science began to take shape in China.

In the 1950s, the Chinese government (2) _____ the National Institute of Pharmaceutical Sciences (NIPS) and the Chinese Academy of Traditional Chinese Medicine (TCM), which played a (3) _____ role in the development of pharmaceutical science in China. In the following (4) _____, China made significant progress in drug discovery and development, with the introduction of new (5) _____ and the establishment of new research institutions.

In recent years, China has become one of the world's leading countries in pharmaceutical research and development. The Chinese government has invested heavily in this field, (6) _____ strong support for both academic research and industrial development. As a result, China has seen (7) _____ in its pharmaceutical industry, with many domestic companies emerging as major players in the global market.

One (8) _____ in the development of pharmaceutical science in China is the successful development of vaccines against COVID-19. Chinese scientists were able to quickly identify the virus and develop (9) _____ , which have been distributed worldwide to help combat the pandemic.

Looking to the future, China is expected to continue its (10) _____ innovation and research in pharmaceutical science, with a particular emphasis on developing new treatments for (11) _____ and rare genetic disorders. With its large population and growing economy, China is well positioned to make (12) _____ to the global pharmaceutical industry in the years to come.

B. Visual Comprehension

Watch a video clip three times and decide whether each of the following statements is true (T) or false (F).

_____ 1. Rihanna Plaza was born with a rare type of tumor inside of her arm.

_____ 2. After 3 days of chemotherapy, the tumor started to shrink.

_____ 3. The FDA approved that drug which treats cancers that all have the same specific tumor mutation.

_____ 4. Less than 3% of tumors have this specific tumor mutation.

_____ 5. Derek Laurie had a cancer that spread throughout his body and recovered within a week of taking the drug.

_____ 6. A drug opens up a new frontier for patients that have this specific mutation.

_____ 7. The video clip shows that cancer treatment targets the specific tumor mutation regardless of a cancer's location.

V. Extended Reading

Read the following dialogue between Dr. Pharmed and students about the history of pharmaceutical development in China, and complete each statement with a proper phrase or sentence given in the box.

Dr. Pharmed: Hello everyone, it's great to have this opportunity to talk about the history of pharmaceutical development in China. I hope you find it as interesting as I do.

Student 1: Thank you for sharing this information with us, Dr. Pharmed. We really appreciate the opportunity to learn more about this topic.

Dr. Pharmed: Absolutely. Pharmaceutical development in China has a rich history that dates back thousands of years. In fact, according to ancient texts, Chinese herbal medicine dates back to the Xia Dynasty, around 2000 BC.

Student 2: That's fascinating. Can you tell us more about the early development of pharmaceuticals in China?

Dr. Pharmed: Absolutely. The early pharmaceuticals in China were mainly based on natural products extracted from plants and animals. Traditional Chinese medicine theory is a core element of the early pharmaceutical development in China, emphasizing the balance and harmony of the body.

Student 3: I'm also interested in the modern history of pharmaceutical development in China. Can you tell us more about that?

Dr. Pharmed: Absolutely. In the modern era, China has made significant progress in pharmaceutical research and development. In the past few decades, China has emerged as one of the largest pharmaceutical markets in the world, with a growing emphasis on innovation and technology.

Student 4: That's impressive. What are some of the recent advancements in Chinese pharmaceuticals?

Dr. Pharmed: In recent years, Chinese pharmaceutical companies have made significant progress in drug discovery, development, and manufacturing. One of the most prominent examples is the development of innovative drugs for diseases such as cancer and hepatitis. Additionally, Chinese companies are also actively involved in international collaboration and innovation, working with global partners to develop new treatment options for patients worldwide.

Student 5: Thank you for sharing this information with us, Dr. Pharmed. It's been a very enlightening conversation and we really appreciate your knowledge and expertise.

Dr. Pharmed: You're welcome, students. I hope you found this discussion as enlightening as I did. Remember, the history of pharmaceutical development in China is a dynamic and exciting field that requires dedication, curiosity, and a passion for knowledge. Keep up the good work and always strive to learn more!

1. Students really _____ about the history of pharmaceutical development in China.

2. Traditional Chinese medicine theory _____.

3. China has _____.

4. Chinese companies have _____, development, and manufacturing.

5. Chinese companies are actively _____.

> A. appreciate the opportunity to learn
> B. made significant progress in drug discovery
> C. emphasizes the balance and harmony of the body
> D. involved in international collaboration and innovation
> E. develop new therapies for cancer patients worldwide
> F. emerged as one of the largest pharmaceutical markets
> G. worked with global partners to develop new treatment options

VI. Topics for Discussion and Essay-writing

1. State one or two notable figures in the history of pharmaceutical development in China that impress you most, and state their contributions to the pharmaceutical development in China.

2. What do you think of the history of pharmaceutical development in China?

3. Talk about significant progress that China has made in pharmaceutical research and development in the modern era.

Chapter II

Basic Knowledge of Drugs

2.1   Drug Classification

Drugs can be classified into different classes based on their chemical structure, **pharmacological** properties, and therapeutic effects. Here are some basic knowledge on drug classes:

Anabolic steroids: These drugs are used to promote muscle growth and repair tissues in the body. They include **testosterone**, **stanozolol**, and **nandrolone**.

Analgesics: These drugs are used to **relieve** pain. They include **acetaminophen**, **ibuprofen**, and **codeine**.

1. How can drugs be classified?

2. How many classes of drugs are mentioned in this section?

3. What are the drugs whose name you are familiar with?

---

pharmacological /ˌfɑːməkəˈlɒdʒɪkl/ *adj*.	药理学的
anabolic /əˈnæbəlɪk/ *adj*.	合成代谢的
steroid /sterɔɪd/ *n*.	类固醇;甾类化合物
testosterone /teˈstɒstərəʊn/ *n*.	睾酮;睾丸素(男性荷尔蒙的一种)
stanozolol /stæˈnɒlɒl/ *n*.	司坦唑醇
nandrolone /ˈnændrəˈləʊn/ *n*.	诺龙(可提高运动成绩的违禁药品)
analgesics /ˌænəlˈdʒɪzɪks/ *n*.	止痛剂;镇痛剂
relieve /rɪˈliːv/ *v*.	缓和;缓解;减轻
acetaminophen /əˌsɪtəˈmɪnəfən/ *n*.	醋氨酚,对乙酰氨基酚(解热镇痛药)
ibuprofen /ˌaɪbjʊˈprəʊfen/ *n*.	布洛芬,异丁苯丙酸(镇痛消炎药)
codeine /ˈkəʊdin/ *n*.	可待因(用于减轻头痛及感冒症状的药物)

Antibiotics: These drugs are used to kill or prevent the growth of **bacteria** that cause infections. They include **penicillin**, **streptomycin**, and **tetracycline**.

Antidepressants: These drugs are used to treat **depression** by altering the levels of **neurotransmitters** in the brain. They include **selective serotonin reuptake inhibitors**(SSRIs), **tricyclic** antidepressants (TCAs), and **monoamine oxidase** inhibitors (MAOIs).

4. What drugs among them have you ever taken before?

Antipsychotics: These drugs are used to treat **schizophrenia**, **bipolar** disorder, and other mental disorders by altering the levels of neurotransmitters in the brain. They include **phenothiazines**, **atypical antipsychotics**, and **clozapines**.

Antihistamines: These drugs are used to treat

5. What are antihistamines

---

bacteria /bæk'tɪrɪə/ n.	细菌
penicillin /ˌpenɪ'sɪlɪn/ n.	青霉素;盘尼西林
streptomycin /ˌstreptə'maɪsɪn/ n.	链霉素
tetracycline /ˌtetrə'saɪklɪn/ n.	四环素
antidepressant /ˌæntɪdɪ'presənt/ n.	抗抑郁剂
depression /dɪ'preʃn/ n.	抑郁;沮丧;不景气
neurotransmitter /'nʊrəʊtrænzmɪtər/ n.	神经递质
selective /sɪ'lektɪv/ adj.	选择性的;有选择的
serotonin /ˌserə'təʊnɪn/ n.	血清素
reuptake /rɪ'ʌpˌteɪk/ n.	重新吸收;重新摄取
inhibitor /ɪn'hɪbɪtə/ n.	抑制剂;抑制者
tricyclic /traɪ'sɪklɪk/ adj.	三环的
monoamine /ˌmɒnəʊr'mɪn/ n.	单胺;一元胺
oxidase /'ɒksədeɪs/ n.	氧化酶
antipsychotics /æntɪpsaɪ'kɒtɪks/ n.	抗精神病药
schizophrenia /ˌskɪtsə'frɪnɪə/ n.	精神分裂症
bipolar /ˌbaɪ'pəʊlər/ adj.	有两极的;双极的
phenothiazine /ˌfɪnəʊ'θaɪəˌzɪn/ n.	吩噻嗪(用作杀虫剂或药物制造)
atypical/eɪ'tɪpɪkəl/ adj.	非典型的
clozapine /k'ləʊzəpaɪn/ n.	[化]氯氮平
antihistamine /ˌæntɪ'hɪstəˌmɪn/ n.	抗组胺药(用于抗过敏)

allergies by blocking **histamine receptors** in the body. They include **diphenhydramine**, **loratadine**, and **cetirizine**.

Antivirals: These drugs are used to treat **viral** infections by **inhibiting** the **replication** of viruses. They include **ribavirin**, **ganciclovir**, and **interferon-alpha**.

Beta-blockers: These drugs are used to treat **hypertension**, heart disease, and other conditions by blocking the action of **adrenaline** on the heart and blood **vessels**. They include **metoprolol**, **atenolol**, and **propranolol**.

Diuretics: These drugs are used to treat high blood pressure by increasing urine production and reducing

used for?

6. What conditions are beta-blockers used to treat?

7. What other drug classes have you learned about in

---

allergy /ˈæləːdʒɪ/ *n.*	过敏反应;过敏症
histamine /ˈhɪstəˌmɪn/ *n.*	组胺
receptor /rɪˈseptər/ *n.*	感受器;受体
diphenhydramine /dɪfenˈhɪdrʌmən/ *n.*	苯海拉明,可他敏(抗过敏药)
loratadine /ləreɪteɪˈdaɪn/ *n.*	氯雷他定(抗组胺药)
cetirizine /sɪˈtɪrɪzɪn/ *n.*	西替利嗪(抗过敏药)
antiviral /ˌæntɪˈvaɪrəl/ *adj.*	抗病毒的
viral /ˈvaɪrəl/ *adj.*	病毒的;病毒引起的
inhibit /ɪnˈhɪbɪt/ *v.*	抑制;禁止;阻止
replication /replɪcation/ *n.*	复制;折叠
ribavirin /ˈraɪbəˌvaɪrɪn/ *n.*	三唑核苷,病毒唑(抗病毒药)
ganciclovir /gænsɪkˈləʊvə/ *n.*	[医]羟甲基无环鸟苷,更昔洛韦
interferon-alpha /ɪntəˈfɪərɒnˈælfə/ *n.*	[医]α-干扰素
beta-blocker /ˈbiːtəbˈlɒkər/ *n.*	[医]β-受体阻滞剂
hypertension /ˌhaɪpərˈtenʃn/ *n.*	高血压
adrenaline /əˈdrenəlɪn/ *n.*	肾上腺素
vessel /ˈvesl/ *n.*	血管;容器;船舰
metoprolol /metɒpˈrɒlɒl/ *n.*	美托洛尔(β-受体阻滞剂)
atenolol /æteˈnɒlɒl/ *n.*	阿替洛尔,氨酰心安(β-受体阻滞剂)
propranolol /prəʊˈprænəˌlɒl/ *n.*	普兰洛尔,心得安(β-受体阻滞剂)
diuretics /daɪˈjʊəretɪks/ *n.*	利尿剂

fluid **retention** in the body. They include **furosemide**, **hydrochlorothiazide**, and **spironolactone**.

These are just a few examples of drug classes. There are many more classes of drugs with varying therapeutic effects and potential side effects.

addition to those mentioned in this section?

2.2 Dosage and Dosage Forms

Dosage refers to the amount of a medication taken by an individual at one time. It is important to follow the recommended dosage as instructed by a healthcare professional to avoid **adverse** effects and achieve the desired therapeutic effect. The dosage may be adjusted based on factors such as age, weight, medical history, and response to the medication.

1. What does dosage refer to?

Dosage form refers to the specific physical or chemical **configuration** in which a medication is presented for **administration**, such as a pill, **capsule**, liquid, or **injection**. The dosage form affects how the medication is absorbed into the body and how it is **metabolized** by the body's

2. What does the dosage form refer to?

3. What can the dosage form affect?

---

retention /rɪˈtenʃn/ n.	保持；保留
furosemide /fjʊˈrəʊsəˌmaɪd/ n.	利尿磺酸；呋喃苯胺酸；利尿灵
hydrochlorothiazide /ˌhaɪdrəˌklɒrəˈθaɪəˌzaɪd/ n.	双氢氯噻嗪，双氢克尿塞（利尿降压药）
spironolactone /spaɪˈrɒnəˈlækˌtəʊn/ n.	螺旋内酯甾酮（利尿药）
dosage /ˈdəʊsɪdʒ/ n.	剂量；用量
adverse /ədˈvɜːrs/ adj.	不利的；有害的；反面的
configuration /kənˌfɪɡjəˈreɪʃn/ n.	安排；布局；格局
administration /ədˌmɪnɪˈstreɪʃn/ n.	施用（药物）；实施；管理
capsule /ˈkæpsl/ n.	胶囊；密封小容器
injection /ɪnˈdʒekʃn/ n.	注射；打针；投入
metabolize /məˈtæbəlaɪz/ v.	使新陈代谢

enzymes. Common drug dosage forms are: **tablets**, capsules, **granules**, injections, eye drops, ear drops, **nasal spray**, oral solution, etc. Different dosage forms may have different effects on the body and may require different methods of administration or **storage**.

4. What common drug dosage forms are mentioned?

When discussing the dosage and dosage forms of a drug, it's important to consider the intended use, the patient's age, weight, and medical history. The following are some common dosage guidelines and forms:

5. What should be taken into account when it comes to the dosage and dosage forms of a drug?

Oral dosage: Many drugs are given orally as tablets, capsules, or liquid **suspensions**. The amount of drug taken is usually measured in milligrams (mg) or **micrograms** (mcg), and the frequency of doses may vary depending on the drug and its intended effect. For example, a single tablet of aspirin may contain 100 mg, while a daily dose of **paracetamol** (acetaminophen) for children may range from 5~10 mg per kilogram of body weight.

6. What forms of drugs does oral dosage include?

Intravenous dosage: Drugs delivered through an intravenous (IV) injection are typically administered by a healthcare professional in a hospital or clinic setting. The dosage form and **concentration** will depend on the drug being used and the patient's condition. For instance, a

7. What is meant by the intravenous dosage?

enzyme /ˈenzaɪm/ n.	酶
tablet /ˈtæblət/ n.	药片;片剂
granule /ˈɡrænjʊl/ n.	颗粒状物;微粒
nasal /neɪzl/ adj.	鼻的;鼻音的
spray /spreɪ/ n.	喷剂;喷雾;水花
storage /ˈstɔːrɪdʒ/ n.	储藏;贮存
suspension /səˈspenʃn/ n.	悬浮;暂停;延缓
microgram /ˈmaɪkrəʊɡræm/ n.	微克(重量单位);百万分之一克
paracetamol /ˌpærəˈsɪtəmɒl/ n.	对乙酰氨基酚,扑热息痛
intravenous /ˌɪntrəˈviːnəs/ adj.	静脉注射的;进入静脉的
concentration /ˌkɒnsnˈtreɪʃn/ n.	浓度;全神贯注;集中

doctor might **administer** a loading dose of **insulin** to a **diabetic** patient before an injection, followed by regular **maintenance** doses throughout the day.

Sublingual dosage: Some drugs can be taken orally as a sublingual tablet or spray. When taken this way, the drug is absorbed directly into the bloodstream through the mouth and throat tissues. The amount of drug taken is usually measured in milligrams (mg) and the frequency of doses may vary depending on the drug and its intended effect. For example, a single tablet of **nicotine patch** may contain 21 mg, while a daily dose of loratadine (a commonly used antihistamine) for allergy symptoms may range from 10 mg to 40 mg per day.

8. What are the advantages of using sublingual dosage?

Topical dosage: Some drugs are applied topically to the skin, muscles, or **mucous membranes**. The amount of drug applied will depend on the product and its intended use. For example, a cream containing **hydrocortisone** may be applied to the affected area once or twice daily, while a topical medication for warts may be applied once a day for several weeks.

9. Have you ever used a certain topical?

It's important to follow the instructions provided by your healthcare provider or pharmacist when taking any medication, including dosage and dosage forms. **Overdosing**

10. Why is it important to follow the instructions when taking any medication?

administer /əd'mɪnɪstər/ v.	施用(药物);管理;施行
insulin /'ɪnsəlɪn/ n.	胰岛素
diabetic /ˌdaɪə'betɪk/ n/adj.	糖尿病患者;糖尿病的
maintenance /'meɪntənəns/ n.	维持;保持;保养
sublingual /sʌb'lɪŋgwəl/ adj.	舌下的;舌下腺的
nicotine patch	尼古丁贴片;戒烟贴
mucous /'mjʊkəs/ adj.	黏液的;黏液覆盖的
membrane /'memˌbreɪn/ n.	膜;薄膜;隔膜
hydrocortisone /ˌhaɪdrə'kɔːtɪzəʊn/ n.	氢化可的松(副肾荷尔蒙之一种)
overdose /'əʊvədəʊs/ n.	过量用药

or **misusing** a drug can lead to serious health **complications**
or adverse effects.

Language Practice

I. Vocabulary Work

*Complete each of the following sentences with a suitable word or expression given
below.*

analgesics	administration	allergy	hypertension
relieve	capsule	receptor	replication
suspension	injection	antiviral	dosage
intravenous	misuse	inhibit	nasal
maintenance	complication	retention	spray

1. _____ is a chronic condition that requires long-term treatment with medication
   to control blood pressure levels.
2. The new _____ drug is effective against a wide range of viruses, including
   influenza and HIV.
3. The patient's recovery has been slowed by a _____ that developed after the
   surgery.
4. The _____ injection of the medication was administered quickly and
   efficiently.
5. The pain medication is designed to _____ the suffering of patients.
6. The antiviral medication works by _____ the replication of the virus in the
   host cell.
7. The doctor recommended that the patient take the _____ with food to reduce
   side effects.
8. The doctor explained that the _____ dose of the medication was crucial for
   the patient's long-term health.

---

misuse /mɪsˈjuːz/ *n.*　　　　　　　使用不当；误用；滥用
complication /ˌkɒmplɪˈkeɪʃn/ *n.*　并发症；使情况复杂化的难题（或困难）

9. The patient must take the medication at the recommended _____ to achieve the desired results.

10. The correct _____ of the medication is crucial for achieving the desired therapeutic effect.

11. The effectiveness of the medication was limited by its poor _____ in the body.

12. The patient's condition worsened due to the _____ of the medication.

13. The doctor recommended that the patient undergo a skin _____ test before starting the new medication.

14. The patient was instructed on how to give himself the _____ at home.

15. The doctor prescribed a _____ for the patient's sore throat.

II. Word Building

Study the Prefixes，Suffixes and Roots in the following grid，and then provide the corresponding word based on the given definition.

Prefixes	Meaning	Example
intra-	"within" or "inside"（在内部；在中间）	intravenous
bi-	"two or having two parts"（二；双；两部分）	bipolar
Suffixes		
-olol	"characteristic of certain beta-blocker medications"（一些β-受体阻滞剂特征的药物）	metoprolol
-ics	"a field of study or a branch of knowledge"（学科或知识领域）	physics
-oid	"a similarity or resemblance to something else"（类似或相似）	steroid
-ological	"a branch of knowledge or a field of study"（知识或学科领域）	pharmacological
Roots		
alg	"pain"（疼，痛）	analgesics
venous	"vein"（静脉）	intravenous

1. a period of two weeks in which an event or activity occurs _____

2. relating to or being blood vessels that carry blood towards the heart _____

3. a type of medication that is used to relieve pain _____
4. relating to the study of living organisms and their interactions with each other and their environment _____
5. relating to the study of society and the interactions between individuals within society _____
6. something that is similar to or resembling the Moon _____
7. a type of medication used to treat bipolar disorder _____
8. relating to communication or awareness within oneself _____
9. the study of matter and energy and how they interact _____
10. the study of numbers, quantities, and their relationships _____

III. Structure & Function

The infinitive phrase "to + verb"（不定式短语）is used to express purpose, intention, or the idea of doing something. For example：

Anabolic steroids are used to promote muscle growth and repair tissues in the body.

Antiviral drugs are used to treat viral infections by inhibiting the replication of viruses.

The infinitive phrase can also function as a subject, object, or complement in a sentence. Here are some examples：

As a subject：

It is important to follow the recommended dosage as instructed by a healthcare professional to avoid adverse effects and achieve the desired therapeutic effect.

As an object：

The company is aiming to introduce a new drug to the market in the next year.

The scientist is trying to identify the active ingredients in the natural medicine.

As a complement：

The pharmacist instructed the customer to take the prescribed medication three times a day.

"To + verb" infinitive phrases are widely used in medical English literature to introduce actions or tasks that need to be performed or completed. This syntax achieves several stylistic effects：

1. Clear and concise expression：The "to＋verb" structure is a common and straightforward way of expressing an action or task. It makes the sentence easy to understand and follow, which is especially important in medical literature where complex information needs to be conveyed clearly and accurately.

2. Emphasis on the action：By using an infinitive phrase, the focus is on the action being described rather than the subject performing it. This can help to emphasize the importance of the task or action, making it more memorable and impactful for readers.

3. Use of future tense：Infinitive phrases often use the future tense, which can help to indicate that the action needs to be done in the future. This can be particularly useful in medical literature, where deadlines or recommendations may need to be given for specific actions to be taken.

4. Contrast with other grammatical structures：The "to＋verb" structure stands out from other grammatical structures such as "-ing" or "-ed" forms, which can create a visual break and draw attention to the action being described. This can be particularly effective in medical literature, where clear and concise language is essential to ensure accurate communication.

Translate each of the following sentences into English.

1. 这家制药公司正在投资研发一种新药,以帮助数百万患者。

_____

_____

2. 科学家工作的主要重点是了解现有药物的作用机制,并提高其治疗性能。

_____

_____

3. 这位科学家正在尝试开发一种新的药物,它将使患者更快地从疾病中康复。

_____

_____

4. 在讨论药物的剂量和剂型时,考虑预期用途、患者年龄、体重和病史是很重要的。

_____

_____

5. 有必要不断监测和评估现有药物的安全性和有效性,以便进行必要的调整或改进。

_____

_____

IV. Audio-visual Exercise

A. Spot Dictation

Listen to a passage twice. Fill in each blank with what you hear while listening.

When taking medication, it is important to follow the dosage recommendations of the doctor or (1) _____ and use the drug forms as recommended to ensure the safety and effectiveness of the medication.

Using medications as recommended is important for several reasons:

1. Effectiveness: When medications are used as (2) _____ , they are more likely to be effective in treating the condition they were intended for. This is because the dosage and frequency of medication have been carefully (3) _____ based on the individual's medical history, age, weight, and other factors.

2. Safety: Overuse or misuse of medications can lead to (4) _____ effects, such as side effects or drug interactions. Using medications as recommended helps to (5) _____ these risks and ensures that patients receive the safest possible treatment.

3. Cost-effectiveness: Using medications as prescribed can also help to reduce healthcare costs (6) _____ . Overuse or misuse of medications can lead to additional medical expenses, such as hospitalizations or emergency room visits, which can (7) _____ by following the recommended treatment plan.

4. Personalized treatment: Each person's (8) _____ are unique, and medications should (9) _____ to their specific condition and circumstances. Using medications as recommended ensures that patients receive personalized treatment that (10) _____ their individual health status

and goals.

In summary, using medications as recommended is essential for achieving (11) _____ , minimizing risks, and ensuring cost-effective and personalized treatment. Patients should always follow the instructions provided by their healthcare provider and never alter their medication regimen without first (12) _____ a healthcare professional.

B. Visual Comprehension

Watch a video clip three times and decide whether each of the following statements is true (T) or false (F).

_____ 1. Aspirin is the most modest product in the medicine cabinet, but may turn out to be the most cost-effective.

_____ 2. Aspirin used for headache or aches is now used for heart attack and stroke prevention.

_____ 3. People who have inherited the gene for Lynch syndrome are at a very high risk for heart attack.

_____ 4. British researchers assume that aspirin might not be without its own potential side effects for colon cancer.

_____ 5. Aspirin may potentially reduce risks for colon cancer, but it has risks for serious gastrointestinal bleeding.

_____ 6. Aspirin has become such a wonder drug that it could cut risks not only for heart attack and stroke, but also for cancer.

_____ 7. Doctors say aspirin can even more dramatically cut risks for colon cancer than colonoscopies.

V. Extended Reading

Read the following dialogue between Dr. Pharmed and students about the classification of pharmaceuticals, and complete the dialogue with a suitable phrase or sentence from the grid.

Dr. Pharmed: Good morning, everyone. Today, I would like to discuss the classification of pharmaceuticals with you.

Student 1: Thank you, Dr. Pharmed. We are curious about how drugs are classified in the pharmaceutical industry.

Dr. Pharmed: The classification of pharmaceuticals is based on their mechanism of action and therapeutic target. ___1___, but the most widely recognized system is the Anatomical Therapeutic Chemical (ATC) system.

Student 2: Can you explain what the ATC system is?

Dr. Pharmed: Sure. The ATC system was developed by the World Health Organization (WHO) and is used to classify drugs according to their therapeutic targets. ___2___: antimicrobials, antivirals, antifungals, antiparasitics, and immunosuppressants. Within each group, drugs are further categorized based on their mechanism of action and therapeutic target.

Student 3: That's interesting. How does the classification of drugs help in drug development?

Dr. Pharmed: ___3___ because it helps researchers identify potential new drugs that have a unique mechanism of action or therapeutic target. It also allows pharmaceutical companies to focus their research efforts on areas where there is a high unmet medical need.

Student 4: What other classification systems are used in the pharmaceutical industry?

Dr. Pharmed: In addition to the ATC system, other classification systems are used in the pharmaceutical industry, such as the International Nonproprietary Name (INN) system and the World Health Organization's Monograph List. ___4___ based on their chemical structure or mechanism of action, respectively.

Student 5: How do these classification systems impact drug development?

Dr. Pharmed: The use of different classification systems can impact drug development in different ways. For example, ___5___, making it easier for doctors and patients to understand how drugs work and what they are intended to treat. On the other hand, the INN system is more specific to chemical structures and can be useful for identifying potential drug candidates based on their chemical properties.

Student 6: Thank you for sharing your knowledge with us, Dr. Pharmed. We appreciate your expertise on this subject.

Dr. Pharmed: You're welcome. Remember, understanding ___6___ and can have a significant impact on patient outcomes. By staying up-to-date on the latest classification systems and trends in pharmaceutical research, we can continue to make progress in improving healthcare worldwide.

_____ 1	A. Drugs are classified into five main groups
_____ 2	B. These systems are used to classify drugs
_____ 3	C. There are different pharmaceutical companies
_____ 4	D. The classification of drugs is important for drug development
_____ 5	E. There are several different classification systems used in the
_____ 6	industry
	F. Drugs can have different classifications based on their mechanisms
	G. the classification of pharmaceuticals is an important aspect of drug development
	H. the ATC system is widely used in clinical practice and regulatory agencies around the world

VI. Topics for Discussion and Essay-writing

1. Give examples to show how drugs are classified.

2. What should be taken into consideration when discussing the dosage and dosage forms of a drug?

3. Why is it important to follow the instructions when taking any medication?

2.3 Drug Actions

Drug actions refer to the physiological effects that a drug has on the body. These effects can be **mediated** by various chemical pathways in the body and can range from therapeutic to **toxic**. Here are some examples of drug actions:

Analgesics: These drugs reduce pain by blocking or inhibiting the **transmission** of pain signals in the nervous system. For example, acetaminophen (paracetamol) works by blocking the enzyme **cytochrome** P450 enzymes in the liver, which reduces the metabolism of other drugs and increases the concentration of acetaminophen in the bloodstream.

Antibiotics: These drugs work by killing or inhibiting the growth of bacteria that cause infections. For example, penicillin works by binding to specific sites on bacterial cell walls and preventing them from forming their own protective structures. This allows the antibiotic to **penetrate** the cell and kill the bacteria.

Antidepressants: These drugs work by altering the levels of neurotransmitters in the brain that regulate mood and emotions. For example, selective serotonin reuptake inhibitors (SSRIs) like fluoxetine work by increasing the

1. What are drug actions?

2. What are the effects of analgesics?

3. How does penicillin kill bacteria?

4. How does fluoxetine work to regulate mood?

---

mediate /ˈmiːdɪeɪt/ v.　　　　　影响;调节;调停
toxic /ˈtɒksɪk/ adj.　　　　　　有毒的;毒性的;中毒的
transmission /trænzˈmɪʃ(ə)n/ n.　　传输;传递;传送
cytochrome /ˈsaɪtəˌkrəʊm/ n.　　　细胞色素
penetrate /ˈpenətreɪt/ v.　　　　穿透;渗入;洞悉

levels of serotonin in the brain, which is involved in regulating mood and reducing symptoms of depression.

Antipsychotics: These drugs work by altering the levels of neurotransmitters in the brain that regulate behavior and thought processes. For example, clozapines work by increasing the levels of **dopamine** in the brain, which is involved in regulating mood and reducing symptoms of schizophrenia.

5. Why can antipsychotics regulate people's behavior and thought processes?

Antihistamines: These drugs work by blocking the action of histamine receptors in the body, which are involved in **allergic** reactions. For example, diphenhydramine works by blocking the action of histamine receptors in the nerve endings, which prevents them from releasing histamine and causing symptoms of an allergic reaction.

6. What type of medicine is diphenhydramine?

These are just a few examples of drug actions. There are many more types of drugs with different mechanisms of action, each with its own unique set of side effects and potential risks.

7. What factors should be taken into account when exploring drug actions?

2.4　Drug Interactions

Drug **interactions** refer to the effects that one drug can have on the activity of another drug when they are taken together. These interactions can be positive, negative, or **neutral**, and can range from mild to severe. Here are some examples of drug interactions:

1. What are drug interactions in general?

---

dopamine /ˈdəʊpəmiːn/ n.　　　　　　多巴胺
allergic /əˈlɜːrdʒɪk/ adj.　　　　　　过敏的;反感的;厌恶的
interaction /ˌɪntərˈækʃ(ə)n/ n.　　　相互作用;互动;沟通
neutral /ˈnjuːtrəl/ adj.　　　　　　　中性的;中立的;暗淡的

Antibiotic-antibiotic **resistance**: When two antibiotics are taken together, they can interact to reduce the effectiveness of both drugs. For example, taking **amoxicillin** (a common antibiotic) with **azithromycin** (another antibiotic) can decrease the **absorption** of amoxicillin in the body and make it less effective against certain bacteria.

Antidepressants and alcohol: Alcohol can increase the **sedative** effects of many antidepressants, leading to increased **drowsiness**, **slurred** speech, and **impaired coordination**. This can also lead to an increased risk of falls and accidents.

Blood thinners and aspirin: Aspirin is a common blood thinner that can increase the risk of bleeding when combined with other blood thinners such as **warfarin** or **heparin**. This can lead to serious complications such as internal **bleeding** or **stroke**.

Diuretics and **lithium**: Lithium is a mood stabilizer that can interact with diuretics (water pills) to increase

2. *Which drug will reduce the body's absorption of amoxicillin?*

3. *What effect does alcohol have on antidepressants?*

4. *What side effect does aspirin have?*

5. *What are the potential side effects of combining diuretics*

---

resistance /rɪ'zɪstəns/ *n*.　　　　　抗药性；抵抗力；阻力
amoxicillin /əˌmɒksɪ'sɪlɪn/ *n*.　　　阿莫西林,羟氨苄青霉(抗生素)
azithromycin /eɪzɪθrə'maɪsɪn/ *n*.　阿奇霉素(抗生素)
absorption /əb'sɔːrpʃ(ə)n/ *n*.　　　吸收；合并；同化
sedative /'sedətɪv/ *adj*.　　　　　　镇静的；有镇静作用的；有催眠作用的
drowsiness /'draʊzinəs/ *n*.　　　　　嗜睡；睡意；昏昏欲睡
slurred /slɜːrd/ *adj*.　　　　　　　　含糊不清的；含含糊糊的；含混的
impair /ɪm'peə/ *v*.　　　　　　　　　损害；削弱；妨碍
coordination /kəʊˌɔːrdɪ'neɪʃ(ə)n/ *n*.　协调；配合；协作
warfarin /'wɔːrfərɪn/ *n*.　　　　　　华法林(血液稀释剂)
heparin /'hepərɪn/ *n*.　　　　　　　肝素(血液稀释剂)
bleeding /'bliːdɪŋ/ *n*.　　　　　　　出血；流血；失血
stroke /strəʊk/ *n*.　　　　　　　　　脑卒中(中风)
lithium /'lɪθɪəm/ *n*.　　　　　　　　锂

urine output and potentially lead to **dehydration** and **electrolyte imbalances**.

with lithium?

Antidepressants and caffeine: Caffeine is a stimulant that can increase **alertness** and energy levels, but when taken with certain antidepressants such as **fluoxetine**, it can increase the risk of **seizures** and muscle **tremors**.

6. With what substance does caffeine have bad effects?

These are just a few examples of drug interactions. It's important for healthcare professionals to be aware of potential drug interactions when prescribing medication to patients, as they can affect the effectiveness of the treatment and increase the risk of side effects and complications.

7. What should be aware of when healthcare professionals prescribe medication to patients?

Language Practice

I. Vocabulary Work

Complete each of the following sentences with a suitable word or expression given below.

mediate	neutral	slurred	dehydration
toxic	resistance	impair	imbalance
penetrate	absorption	coordination	alertness
allergic	sedative	bleeding	seizure
interaction	drowsiness	stroke	transmission

1. The drug is designed to _____ the blood-brain barrier, allowing it to

dehydration /ˌdiːhaɪˈdreɪʃ(ə)n/ *n.*   脱水;干燥;失水
electrolyte /ɪˈlektrəlaɪt/ *n.*   电解质;电解液
imbalance /ɪmˈbæləns/ *n.*   失衡;失调;不安定
alertness /əˈlɜːrtnəs/ *n.*   警觉;警戒;机敏
fluoxetine /fluːˈɒksəˌtiːn/ *n.*   氟西汀(抗抑郁药)
seizure /ˈsiːʒər/ *n.*   癫痫;疾病突然发作
tremor /ˈtremər/ *n.*   颤抖;战栗;哆嗦

effectively treat conditions affecting the central nervous system.

2. The drug blocks the _____ of signals between nerve cells, which can help alleviate symptoms of conditions such as anxiety and depression.

3. Patients taking _____ medications should inform their doctor before starting any new drugs, as some interactions can lead to dangerous side effects.

4. The interaction between these two drugs is considered _____ , meaning that they can be used together without any significant concerns about adverse effects.

5. Patients taking this drug should avoid alcohol and other _____ substances, as they can interact and worsen the effects of the medication.

6. _____ reactions to the medication can range from mild to severe, so it's important to monitor any symptoms closely and seek medical attention if necessary.

7. Certain pain relievers, such as aspirin or ibuprofen, can interact with blood thinners and increase the risk of stroke in patients who have had a previous _____ .

8. Some drug interactions can lead to excessive _____ and respiratory depression, which can be life-threatening in some cases.

9. Patients undergoing surgery or other invasive procedures may be advised to stop taking certain medications that can increase the risk of _____ , in order to minimize complications during and after the procedure.

10. Some patients may develop _____ to certain medications over time, which can make it more difficult to effectively treat their condition and require alternative drug therapies.

11. The combination of this medication with other drugs that _____ cognitive function can increase the risk of side effects such as dizziness and confusion.

12. Some drug interactions can increase the rate of _____ of certain medications, leading to higher levels of the active ingredient in the blood and potentially dangerous side effects.

13. Researchers are investigating how the medication can _____ the response of cancer cells to chemotherapy.

14. This medication can cause _____ speech as a side effect, which may indicate that the patient is experiencing an adverse reaction to the drug.

15. The combination of this medication with other drugs that cause _____ can increase the risk of adverse effects such as dry mouth and constipation.

II. Word Building

Study the Prefixes，Suffixes and Roots in the following grid，and then provide the corresponding word based on the given definition.

Prefixes	Meaning	Example
cyto-	"cell"（细胞）	cytochrome
de-	"away," "remove" or "reverse"（离开；去除）	dehydration
Suffixes		
-ness	"the quality, a state or condition"（性质；状态或情况）	alertness
-arin	used in the names of certain drugs or chemicals to indicate their origin or chemical structure（用于一些药物或化学物名后表明其化学结构来源）	warfarin
-illin	characteristic of certain antibiotics（一些抗生素特征的药物）	amoxicillin
-etine	characteristic of certain antidepressants（一些抗抑郁药物）	fluoxetine
Roots		
chrom(o)	"color" or "pigment"（颜色或色素）	cytochrome
electr(o)	"electricity"（电）	electrolyte

1. a type of anticoagulant medication that is used to prevent blood clots from forming _____

2. a type of antibiotic that is used to treat bacterial infections _____

3. to become worse or less effective over time, typically as a result of neglect or damage _____

4. a quality or state of being gentle, affectionate, and caring towards others

   _____

5. a structure made of DNA and protein found in the nucleus of cells, which carries genetic information in the form of genes _____

6. a test that records the electrical activity of the heart over a period of time using electrodes attached to the skin _____

7. the jelly-like substance within a cell, in which the cell's organelles are suspended

   _____

8. the scientific study of the structure, function, and evolution of the cell _____

9. to kill or injure someone by passing an electric current through their body

_____

10. a tricyclic antidepressant medication that is used to treat major depressive disorder

_____

III. Structure & Function

Gerund phrases（动名词短语）are widely used structures in English for medical purposes. They can be used as subject, object, predicative, attribute and adverbial modifiers to convey complex ideas and actions. For example：

Testing new drugs is essential in determining their safety and efficacy.

Doctors recommend avoiding strenuous exercise after surgery.

The main concern is controlling the spread of infection.

The waiting room was filled with anxious patients.

Despite experiencing side effects, she continued with the medication.

The hospital is equipped with state-of-the-art facilities for treating patients.

The risk of bleeding is associated with taking these medications.

Gerund structures are widely used in English for medical purposes because they provide a concise and efficient way to describe processes, actions, or states that are being studied or described. By using gerunds, English speakers can quickly and clearly communicate the subject of the action or process without having to create complex sentences or use multiple words to describe it.

In science and medicine, concise and efficient communication is crucial. Researchers and doctors need to quickly and accurately convey information about experiments, treatments, diseases, and other topics related to their fields. By using gerund structures, they can easily and effectively communicate this information without having to rely on cumbersome sentence structures or extra words that might clutter their messages.

Additionally, gerund structures are particularly useful in technical writing because they allow the writer to highlight the subject of the action or process being described. This emphasis on the subject helps readers quickly understand the main point being made and can improve the flow of information in a document or report.

Translate each of the following sentences into English.

1. 识别新的治疗靶点对于开发新药至关重要。

_____

_____

2. 研究人员发现该药物在缩小肿瘤方面有效。

_____

_____

3. 这项研究的主要目的是评估新化合物的安全性和有效性。

_____

_____

4. 青霉素通过结合细菌细胞壁上的特定位点来发挥作用,阻止它们形成自身的保护结构。

_____

_____

5. 同时服用阿莫西林和阿奇霉素可能降低阿莫西林在体内的吸收,从而降低其对某些细菌的有效性。

_____

_____

IV. Audio-visual Exercise

A. Spot Dictation

Listen to a passage twice. Fill in each blank with what you hear while listening.

Drug actions and effects on the body are complex and multifaceted. Drugs can act on (1) _____ physiological systems, including the nervous system, cardiovascular system, respiratory system, digestive system, and (2) _____ system.

When a drug is ingested or injected, it interacts with specific receptors in the body, leading to a cascade of (3) _____ reactions that ultimately result in its therapeutic or adverse effects. The type and severity of these effects depend on several factors, including the drug's chemical (4) _____ , potency, route of administration, duration of use, and individual differences in (5) _____ and sensitivity.

For example, some drugs can stimulate or inhibit the activity of (6) _____,
which are chemical messengers that transmit signals between nerve cells. This can
lead to a range of effects on mood, cognition, and behavior, such as sedation,
stimulation, depression, or anxiety.

Other drugs can affect the heart (7) _____, blood pressure, and
fluid balance, either by increasing or decreasing their levels. This can have (8) _____
_____ for cardiovascular health and overall well-being, especially in
individuals with pre-existing conditions or (9) _____.

Drugs can also affect the respiratory system by altering lung function and
oxygenation. Some drugs can cause (10) _____ or paralysis, while
others can increase airway resistance or inflammation.

In addition to their (11) _____ on physiological systems, drugs
can also have indirect effects through interactions with other drugs or substances.
For example, alcohol can enhance the sedative effects of some medications, while
certain drugs can impair (12) _____ and increase the risk of bleeding
or organ damage.

B. Visual Comprehension

*Watch a video clip three times and decide whether each of the following
statements is true (T) or false (F).*

_____ 1. A panel of doctors warned that every drug in medicine cabinets in
America is not safe.

_____ 2. The panel said the recommended dosage level of acetaminophen
products should be lowered.

_____ 3. Drug safety experts recommended lowering the maximum dose of
over-the-counter acetaminophen products to 1000 milligrams.

_____ 4. The FDA official said families need make sure they know whether it's
a prescription product or an over-the-counter product.

_____ 5. Acetaminophen is also an ingredient in many other over-the-counter
medicines.

_____ 6. Each year 458 deaths from liver failure in the U. S. are due to acetaminophen overdose.

_____ 7. The makers of Tylenol said that new regulations could actually reduce serious side effects.

V. Extended Reading

Read the following dialogue between Dr. Pharmed and students about drug interactions and contraindications, and choose the best answer to each question according to the dialogue.

Dr. Pharmed: Hello everyone, it's great to have this opportunity to talk about drug interactions and contraindications. I hope you find it as interesting as I do.

Student 1: Thank you for sharing this information with us, Dr. Pharmed. We really appreciate the opportunity to learn more about this topic.

Dr. Pharmed: Absolutely. Drug interactions and contraindications are important aspects of pharmacy that require careful attention. Drug interactions occur when two or more drugs interact with each other to produce a pharmacodynamic or pharmacokinetic effect that is different from the individual drugs.

Student 2: That's fascinating. Can you give us some examples of drug interactions?

Dr. Pharmed: Absolutely. One example of drug interactions is the interaction between warfarin and aspirin. Warfarin is an anticoagulant that reduces blood clotting, while aspirin is a nonsteroidal anti-inflammatory drug that also reduces blood clotting. When warfarin and aspirin are taken together, the risk of bleeding increases, which can be life-threatening in some cases.

Student 3: I'm also interested in contraindications. Can you tell us more about those?

Dr. Pharmed: Absolutely. Contraindications refer to situations in which a drug should not be used because it can cause serious harm to the patient's health. For example, NSAIDs such as ibuprofen and naproxen are contraindicated in patients with ulcers or gastritis because they can increase the risk of bleeding ulcers and worsen gastritis symptoms. Another example is the use of aspirin in patients with asthma because it can trigger bronchospasms and worsen asthma symptoms.

Student 4: That's very interesting. How do we prevent drug interactions and contraindications?

Dr. Pharmed: Drug interactions and contraindications can be prevented by several measures. One important measure is to understand the drugs being taken by the patient and their potential interactions and contraindications with other drugs or conditions. It is also important to provide the patient with complete information about their prescribed drugs, including potential side effects and interactions, so they can make informed decisions about their medication usage. Another measure is to maintain accurate records of all medication given to ensure coordination between health professionals, avoid duplicate prescriptions, and detect potential drug interactions or contraindications. Finally, it is important to remain vigilant for potential drug interactions or contraindications when prescribing new drugs or monitoring patients on medication therapy.

Student 5: Thank you for sharing this information with us, Dr. Pharmed. It's been a very enlightening conversation and we really appreciate your knowledge and expertise.

Dr. Pharmed: You're welcome. I hope you found this discussion as enlightening as I did. Remember, drug interactions and contraindications are a crucial aspect of pharmacy that require constant vigilance and attention. Keep up the good work and always strive to learn more!

1. Two or more drugs may interact with each other to produce _____ .

   A. an effect different from the individual drugs

   B. a side effect for patients who take them

   C. an adverse effect on patients' condition

   D. a reduced effect of the drugs combined

2. What is the effect of warfarin and aspirin taken together?

    A. It causes serious drug interactions.

    B. It reduces the risk of blood clotting.

    C. It increases the risk of bleeding.

    D. It has no effect on blood clotting.

3. Aspirin should be contraindicated in patients with ulcers or gastritis because it can _____ .

    A. trigger bronchospasms and worsen asthma symptoms

    B. increase the risk of developing ulcers or gastritis

    C. increase the risk of bleeding ulcers and gastritis

    D. cause serious harm to the patient's health

4. Which of the following is NOT an effective way to prevent drug interactions and contraindications?

    A. Maintaining accurate records of all medication given to patients.

    B. Providing the patient with partial information about their drugs.

    C. Remaining vigilant for potential drug interactions or contraindications.

    D. Understanding the drugs' potential interactions and contraindications.

5. Which of the following statements is not true of drug interactions and contraindications?

    A. They can be prevented in several ways.

    B. They can result in serious harm to the patient.

    C. They require constant vigilance and attention.

    D. They occur only when new drugs are prescribed.

VI. Topics for Discussion and Essay-writing

1. Please explain briefly to patients what are drug actions.

2. What are drug interactions?

3. Why is it important to be aware of potential drug interactions when taking medication?

2.5 Drug Contraindications

Drug **contraindications** refer to conditions or diseases in which the use of a specific drug is inappropriate or potentially harmful. Contraindications can occur in various situations, including interactions with other drugs, allergies or **hypersensitivity** to the drug, and specific diseases or conditions that make it difficult to use the drug safely.

Some common drug contraindications include:

Drug interactions: certain drugs may interact with other drugs to produce adverse reactions or side effects. For example, taking aspirin and ibuprofen together can increase the risk of bleeding, while certain antibiotics can reduce the effectiveness of birth control pills.

Allergies and hypersensitivity: certain drugs may cause allergic reactions or hypersensitivity reactions in some people, such as penicillin allergy, aspirin-induced asthma, and so on.

Specific diseases or conditions: some drugs may not be suitable for people with specific diseases or conditions. For example, beta-blockers may not be suitable for people with heart failure or asthma, while NSAIDs may not be suitable for people with **ulcerative colitis** or heart disease.

Pregnancy and **lactation**: certain drugs may be harmful

1. What are drug contra-indications?

2. What do drug interactions mean?.

3. What do two examples show?

---

contraindication /ˌkɒntrəˌɪndɪˈkeɪʃn/ n.　　禁忌征候
hypersensitivity /ˌhaɪpəˌsensəˈtɪvətɪ/ n.　　超敏反应;过敏性反应
ulcerative /ˈʌlsərətɪv/ adj.　　溃疡(性)的
colitis /kəˈlaɪtɪs/ n.　　结肠炎
pregnancy /ˈpregnənsɪ/ n.　　怀孕;妊娠;丰富
lactation /lækˈteʃən/ n.　　哺乳期

to pregnant women or **breastfeeding** mothers, and may even affect the **fetus** or nursing baby. For example, **tetracyclines** are **contraindicated** during pregnancy, while some NSAIDs are not recommended for breastfeeding mothers.

Age: certain drugs may not be suitable for children or elderly people due to differences in their body structure and function. For example, NSAIDs may cause **kidney** damage in children and elderly people, while aspirin is not recommended for children under 12 years old due to the risk of **Reye's syndrome**.

Comorbidities: certain drugs may not be suitable for patients with certain comorbidities, such as diabetes, hypertension, liver disease, kidney disease, and other chronic diseases. It is important to **consult** with your doctor before using any medication to ensure its safety and effectiveness based on your specific health condition.

4. Why are certain drug not recommended during pregnancy and lactation?

5. Why is age an important consideration as to drug contraindications?

6. How can comorbidities affect the suitability of certain drugs for patients?

2.6 Drug Metabolism

Drug metabolism refers to the biological chemical processes that occur in the body after a drug is administered and transformed into a different form. These processes

1. What are the main processes involved in drug metabolism?

---

breastfeeding /brest'fidɪŋ/ v. 用母乳喂养;哺乳
fetus /'fiːtəs/ n. 胎;胎儿
tetracycline /ˌtetrə'saɪklɪn/ 四环素
contraindicate /ˌkɒntrə'ɪndɪkeɪt/ v. 显示(治疗或处置)不当;禁忌(药物或疗法)
kidney /'kɪdnɪ/ n. 肾;肾脏
Reye's syndrome 雷依氏综合征
comorbidity /kəmɔː'bɪdətɪ/ n. 合并症
consult /kən'sʌlt/ v. 咨询;商量;查阅

include **hydrolysis**, **oxidation**, reduction, and **conjugation**.

Hydrolysis is a biological chemical reaction that occurs in the body and involves the addition of a water **molecule** to a molecule or a salt to **split** a chemical **bond**. In drug metabolism, hydrolysis is an important process that can **convert** drugs into inactive or less active **metabolites**. Hydrolysis can be **catalyzed** by enzymes or acid/base conditions in the body. For example, aspirin can be **hydrolyzed** to **salicylic** acid by **esterases**.

2. *How does hydrolysis occur in drug metabolism?*

Oxidation is a biological chemical reaction that involves the loss of a **hydrogen** atom or a negative charge from a molecule or a salt to form a more highly reactive chemical species. In drug metabolism, oxidation is an important process that can convert drugs into more active or less active metabolites. Oxidation is usually catalyzed by enzymes such as cytochrome P450. For example, **dextromethorphan** can be **oxidized** to **dextrorphan** by CYP2D6.

3. *What role does oxidation play in drug metabolism?*

Reduction is one of the three main pathways for drug

4. *How does reduction*

---

hydrolysis /haɪˈdrɒlɪsɪs/ *n*.	水解	
oxidation /ɒksɪˈdeʃən/ *n*.	氧化	
conjugation /kɒndʒəˈgeɪʃn/ *n*.	结合	
molecule /ˈmɒlɪkjuːl/ *n*.	分子;微小颗粒	
split /splɪt/ *v*./*n*.	分裂;分开;裂缝	
bond /bɒnd/ *n*.	纽带;联系	
convert /kənˈvɜːrt/ *v*.	(使)转变;改造	
metabolite /meˈtæbəˌlaɪt/ *n*.	代谢物	
catalyze /ˈkætlˌaɪz/ *vt*.	催化;促进	
hydrolyze /ˈhaɪdrəˌlaɪz/ *n*.	水解	
salicylic /ˌsæləˈsɪlɪk/ *adj*.	水杨酸的	
esterase /ˈestəˌreɪs/ *n*.	酯酶	
hydrogen /ˈhaɪdrədʒən/ *n*.	氢	
dextromethorphan /dekstrəʊmɪˈθɔːfn/ *n*.	右美沙芬	
oxidize /ˈɒksɪdaɪz/ *v*.	使氧化;使生锈	
dextrorphan /ˈdekstrɔːfn/ *n*.	右啡烷;右羟吗喃	

metabolism. It involves the reduction of **carbonyl** groups in the drug molecule, resulting in the formation of new compounds with different pharmacological properties. Here are examples of drugs that undergo reduction:

Acetaminophen: Acetaminophen is metabolized to several **derivatives**, including acetyl-CoA and **acetylcholine**, which have little or no effect on the body. However, some of these metabolites are also converted to other drugs such as **benzodiazepines**, which can have adverse effects.

Ibuprofen: Ibuprofen is metabolized to several derivatives, including **ibuprofenone** and **naproxenone**, which have similar pharmacological properties to ibuprofen but may have different side effects.

Diphenhydramine: Diphenhydramine is metabolized to form **dextroamphetamine**, which has **psychoactive** properties and can cause **addiction** and **withdrawal** symptoms when taken in high doses.

Conjugation is a biological chemical reaction that involves the combination of two or more molecules through a linkage such as an **ester**, **glucuronide**, or **sulfate** group.

occur in drug metabolism?

5. How does conjugation

---

carbonyl /ˈkɑːbənɪl/ n.	碳酰基；羰基
derivative /dɪˈrɪvətɪv/ n./adj.	派生物
acetylcholine /ˌæsətɪlˈkəʊliːn/ n.	乙酰胆碱
benzodiazepine /ˌbenzəʊdaɪˈeɪzɪpiːn/ n.	苯(并)二氮(用于制造各种镇静药)
ibuprofenone /ˈaɪbjʊˈprɒfən/ n.	与布洛芬相关的衍生物
naproxenone /nəˈprɒksən/ n.	与萘普列克松相关的化合物
diphenhydramine /dɪfenˈhɪdrʌmən/	苯海拉明，可他敏(抗过敏药)
dextroamphetamine /ˌdekstrəʊæmˈfetəmɪn/ n.	右旋安非他命
psychoactive /ˌsaɪkəʊˈæktɪv/ adj.	对精神起作用的；影响精神行为的
addiction /əˈdɪkʃn/ n.	毒瘾；着迷；嗜好
withdrawal /wɪðˈdrɔːəl/ n.	撤回；退出
ester /ˈestər/ n.	酯
glucuronide /glʊˈkjʊərənaɪd/ n.	葡(萄)糖苷酸
sulfate /ˈsʌlˌfeɪt/ n.	硫酸盐

In drug metabolism, conjugation is an important process that can convert drugs into more water-soluble metabolites for easier **excretion** from the body. Conjugation can be catalyzed by enzymes such as UDP-**glucuronyltransferase** or **sulfotransferase**. For example, morphine can be conjugated with **glucuronic** acid to form **morphine**-3-glucuronide, which is more water-soluble and can be easily excreted from the body.

contribute to drug metabolism?

Drug metabolism can result in the drug becoming more or less active or even toxic. Therefore, the metabolism of drugs is crucial for determining their **efficacy** and safety.

Language Practice

I. Vocabulary Work

Complete each of the following sentences with a suitable word or expression given below.

contraindication	comorbidity	convert	derivative
hypersensitivity	consult	metabolite	psychoactive
efficacy	oxidation	hydrogen	addiction
lactation	conjugation	split	withdrawal
kidney	molecule	bond	excretion

1. The _____ of this medication with another compound enhances its bioavailability and efficacy.

2. The active ingredient in this medication is a _____ of a naturally occurring

---

excretion /ɪkˈskrɪʃən/ *n*.   （动植物的）排泄；排泄物
glucuronyltransferase /ɡljuːˈkʊərənɪltrænsfrəz/ *n*.   葡糖醛酸基转移酶
sulfotransferase /sʌlfətrænsfˈreɪz/ *n*.   转磺酶；磺基转移酶
glucuronic /gluːˈkjʊərənɪk/ *adj*.   葡糖醛酸
morphine /ˈmɔːfin/ *n*.   吗啡
efficacy /ˈefɪkəsɪ/ *n*.   功效；效力

compound.

3. The old lady exhibited _____ to the medication and required immediate treatment.

4. The patient's _____ with diabetes mellitus requires special consideration when prescribing medication.

5. The _____ of the new medication in treating the condition has been well-documented in clinical trials.

6. The medication contains a chemical bond between a carbon atom and a _____ atom, which is essential for its bioactivity.

7. The professor prescribed a medication that forms a _____ with the receptors in the patient's body, effectively treating the condition.

8. The patient's current health condition is a _____ to the use of this medication.

9. The gentleman has a history of _____ to pain medication and requires special monitoring when prescribed similar medications.

10. The _____ of the active ingredient in the medication can lead to its degradation and reduced efficacy.

11. The drug is not recommended for use during _____ due to potential effects on milk production and quality.

12. The police officer was admitted to the hospital due to _____ symptoms after abruptly stopping the prescribed medication.

13. The substance is _____ and should only be used under the supervision of a healthcare professional.

14. The _____ of this medication may accumulate in the body and cause side effects.

15. The doctor recommended that the patient _____ from tablets to liquid medication due to difficulty in swallowing.

II. Word Building

Study the Prefixes, Suffixes and Roots in the following grid, and then provide the corresponding word based on the given definition.

Prefixes	Meaning	Example
hyper-	"excessive" or "greater than normal" (过分;大于正常)	hypersensitivity
oxi-	"oxygen" (氧;氧气)	oxidation
Suffixes		
-itis	"inflammation or swelling" (发炎;肿)	colitis
Roots		
ulcerate	"to have or form an ulcer" (形成溃疡)	ulcerative
contra	"against" or "opposite of" (反对;相反)	contraindication
morbid	"sick or diseased" (生病的)	comorbidity
hydro	"water" or "related to water" (水;与水有关的)	hydrolysis
psycho	"mind" or "psyche" (精神;心理)	psychoactive

1. excessively active or energetic _____

2. a substance that combines with another substance to produce an oxide

_____

3. inflammation of the joints _____

4. inflammation of the appendix _____

5. the process of becoming ulcerated; the state of being ulcerated _____

6. to violate or act in opposition to a law, rule, or agreement _____

7. the prevention of conception or impregnation _____

8. the quality of being morbid; excessive preoccupation with gloomy or gruesome thoughts _____

9. relating to or involving the use of water power to generate electricity _____

10. a mental disorder characterized by profound disturbances in thought, perception, and behavior _____

III. Structure & Function

In English the conjunction "while" is often used to express a contrasting idea. It compares two different statements or situations, indicating that they are opposite or in opposition to each other. For example:

Beta blockers may not be suitable for people with heart failure or asthma, __*while*__ *NSAIDs* (非类固醇消炎药) *may not be suitable for people with ulcerative* *colitis or heart disease.*

NSAIDs may cause kidney damage in children and elderly people, <u>while</u> aspirin is not recommended for children under 12 years old due to the risk of Reye's syndrome.

A contrasting idea can be expressed in many other ways such as **whereas, in contrast to, by contrast, by comparison, in comparison to, on the other hand, however, conversely, unlike,** etc.. For example:

<u>Whereas</u> aspirin is known to thin the blood and reduce pain, ibuprofen can increase the risk of bleeding, thus creating a drug interaction that can be harmful.

<u>In contrast to</u> aspirin, nonsteroidal anti-inflammatory drugs (NSAIDs) should not be used by patients with a history of stomach ulcers or bleeding disorders.

<u>By comparison to</u> other anticoagulants, warfarin has a higher risk of food and drug interactions that can affect its efficacy and safety.

<u>By contrast</u>, the interaction between aspirin and certain pain medications can lead to an increase in side effects, such as stomach bleeding or drowsiness.

<u>On the other hand</u>, some drugs can interact with each other and cause adverse effects that may be harmful to patients.

<u>Conversely</u>, even if a drug is generally considered safe, it may still have interactions with other medications that could be harmful.

<u>Unlike</u> individuals with no medical conditions, patients with specific health issues may be more susceptible to drug interactions and contraindications, requiring closer attention from healthcare providers.

Translate the following sentences, using in each an expression given in parentheses.

1. 与一些可以随餐服用的药物不同,某些药物必须空腹服用以确保正确吸收和有效性。(unlike)

_____

_____

2. 同时服用阿司匹林和布洛芬会增加出血的风险,而某些抗生素则会降低避孕药的有效性。(while)

3. 相比之下,重要的是要注意,并非所有的药物相互作用都是有害的;在某些情况下,有些甚至可能是有益的。(by contrast)

4. 尽管许多人认为同时使用多种药物是有益的,但了解可能导致严重健康问题的潜在药物相互作用是很重要的。(whereas)

5. 对于医疗专业人员来说,仔细考虑药物相互作用和禁忌证非常重要,反之,如果不这样做,可能导致患者出现严重的并发症。(on the other hand)

IV. Audio-visual Exercise

A. Sentence Dictation

Please listen to each sentence twice. First listening is for you to understand the general meaning of the sentence. Try to repeat the sentence after you listen to it for a second time, and then write down the whole sentence during the pauses. You'll listen to all the sentences for a third time for checking your dictation.

1. Drug metabolism

2. Certain drugs

3. Drug contraindications

4. Certain drugs

5. It is important to

B. Visual Comprehension

Watch a video clip three times and decide whether each of the following statements is true（T）or false（F）.

_____ 1. The LA Court released documents about the cause of Michael Jackson's death.

_____ 2. The documents were released 12 months after Michael Jackson's shocking death.

_____ 3. Toxicology（毒理）analysis showed that Michael Jackson had lethal levels of propofol（二异丙酚）in his blood.

_____ 4. Propofol is a powerful anesthetic（麻醉药）intended for use at home.

_____ 5. Jackson had reportedly been using propofol at home for years to battle his stomach pain.

_____ 6. Los Angeles police didn't believe it was legal for Dr. Murray to use propofol.

_____ 7. The criminal defense attorney Darren Kavinoky said Michael Jackson's death was criminal negligence.

V. Extended Reading

Read the following dialogue between Dr. Pharmed and students about drug metabolism, and complete each statement with a proper phrase or sentence given in the box.

Dr. Pharmed：Good morning, everybody. Today, we will be discussing drug metabolism.

Student 1：Thank you, Dr. Pharmed. We are eager to learn more about how drugs are metabolized in the body.

Dr. Pharmed：Drug metabolism is the process by which drugs are broken down and eliminated from the body. It involves a series of enzymatic reactions that take place in various organs and tissues throughout the body. The rate at which drugs are metabolized can vary depending on factors such as age, sex, weight, and genetics.

Student 2：Can you explain the two main types of drug metabolism?

Dr. Pharmed: Yes, there are two main types of drug metabolism: bioavailability and first-pass effect. Bioavailability refers to the extent to which a drug is absorbed into the bloodstream after it is administered. This can be influenced by factors such as the route of administration, dose, and individual differences in drug metabolism. First-pass effect, on the other hand, refers to the metabolic breakdown of drugs that occurs before they reach their target cells. These drugs may be metabolized by enzymes in the liver or other organs, leading to a decrease in their concentration in the bloodstream.

Student 3: What happens to drugs that are not metabolized properly?

Dr. Pharmed: Drugs that are not metabolized properly can have a variety of negative effects on patients. For example, if a drug is not metabolized quickly enough, it may build up in the bloodstream and cause toxicity or adverse effects. Additionally, drugs that are not metabolized properly may not be effective at all, leading to treatment failure. As pharmacologists, it's important for us to understand how drugs are metabolized in order to develop effective treatment plans and monitor patient outcomes.

Student 4: Thank you for explaining this complex topic to us, Dr. Pharmed. We feel much more prepared to discuss it with our future patients.

Dr. Pharmed: You're welcome. Remember, drug metabolism is an important aspect of drug therapy and plays a crucial role in ensuring safe and effective treatment of patients. By staying informed and consulting with healthcare providers, we can help ensure that our patients receive the best possible care.

1. Drug metabolism is _____ .
2. The rate at which drugs are metabolized can vary _____ .
3. Bioavailability can be influenced by factors such as _____ .
4. First-pass effect, on the other hand, _____ that occurs before they reach their target cells.
5. Drug metabolism is an important aspect of drug therapy and plays a crucial role _____ .

A. how drugs are metabolized in the body

B. refers to the metabolic breakdown of drugs

C. in ensuring safe and effective treatment of patients

D. depending on factors such as age, sex, weight, and genetics

E. take place in various organs and tissues throughout the body

F. the process by which drugs are broken down and eliminated from the body

G. the route of administration, dose, and individual differences in drug metabolism

VI. Topics for Discussion and Essay-writing

1. What are drug contraindications? Under what circumstances may the contraindications occur?

2. Why is it essential for healthcare providers to carefully consider drug contraindications when prescribing drugs to patients?

3. What is drug metabolism? What does it do to a drug efficacy?

Chapter III

Research and Development of Drugs

3.1 The Basic Process of Drug Research and Development

The process of drug research and development typically involves a series of steps aimed at discovering, developing, and **commercializing** compounds with the potential to treat human diseases. The process is complex and costly, typically taking 10 to 15 years and millions of dollars to bring a new drug to market. The following is a general description of the drug research and development process:

1. What is said about the process of drug research and development?

Target Identification: The first step in drug research and development is to identify a target that is associated with a particular disease. This target can be a **protein**, gene, or other **biomolecule** that plays a role in the

2. What is the first step in drug research and development?

commercialize /kəˈmɜːʃlaɪz/ v.	使商业化；以……利
target /ˈtɑːrgɪt/ n.	靶子；目标；对象
identification /aɪˌdentɪfɪˈkeɪʃn/ n.	识别；鉴定；确认
protein /ˈprəʊtiːn/ n.	蛋白质
biomolecule /baɪəmɒˈlɪkjuːl/ n.	生物分子

disease process.

Drug **Screening**: Once a target is identified, **high-throughput** screening（HTS）techniques are typically used to **evaluate** thousands or millions of compounds to identify those that show promise as potential drug candidates. These compounds can come from natural sources, **synthetic** libraries, or virtual libraries.

3. What is the purpose of drug screening?

Lead Identification: After screening, the compounds that show the most promise as drug **candidates** are selected for further **evaluation**. This is called lead identification. The goal is to identify one or more leads that have the best combination of **potency**, **selectivity**, **pharmacokinetics**, and safety.

4. What does lead identification mean?

Lead Optimization: Once lead compounds are identified, they undergo a series of chemical modifications to improve their potency, selectivity, stability, and pharmacokinetic properties. This process is called lead **optimization** and aims to identify the "best-in-class" drug candidate.

5. Why is there a process called lead optimization?

Preclinical Trials: The drug candidate is then evaluated in **preclinical trials** to assess its safety and efficacy in

---

screening /ˈskriːnɪŋ/ n.	筛选;筛查	
high-throughput /haɪ ˈθruːˌpʊt/ n.	高流量	
evaluate /ɪˈvæljʊeɪt/ v.	评估;评价	
synthetic /sɪnˈθetɪk/ adj.	合成的;人造的	
candidate /ˈkændɪdət/ n.	候选人;应试者;适合……的人/物	
evaluation /ɪˌvæljʊˈeɪʃn/ n.	评估;评价	
potency /ˈpəʊtnsɪ/ n.	效力;药力;药效	
selectivity /sɪˌlekˈtɪvɪtɪ/ n.	选择性;专一性	
pharmacokinetics /ˌfɑːməkəʊkaiˈnetɪks/ n.	药物(代谢)动力学	
optimization /ˈɒptəmaɪˈzeɪʃən/ n.	最佳化;最优化;优选法	
preclinical /prɪˈklɪnɪkəl/ adj.	临床应用前的;潜伏期的	
trial /ˈtraɪəl/ n.	试验;试用;审讯	

animal models of the disease. These trials also help to establish the **pharmacodynamic** properties of the drug candidate and identify any potential side effects or **toxicities**.

6. *What is the purpose of preclinical trials?*

Clinical Trials：After preclinical trials are successful, the drug candidate enters clinical trials, which are divided into three phases：Phase I, Phase II, and Phase III. Phase I trials evaluate the safety of the drug candidate in humans, including any potential side effects or adverse reactions at different doses. Phase II trials evaluate the efficacy of the drug candidate in patients with the target disease and further assess its safety **profile** in a larger patient population. Phase III trials involve a larger patient population to further **validate** the safety and efficacy of the drug candidate and establish its long-term effects.

7. *How many phases are clinical trials divided into? What is each phase used for?*

Regulatory Approval：If successful completion of Phase III trials is achieved, the drug candidate typically receives regulatory approval from the Food and Drug Administration（FDA）or other regulatory agencies worldwide for **commercialization** and use in patients.

Post-Approval **Monitoring**：After regulatory approval is **granted**, post-approval monitoring occurs to ensure the safety and efficacy of the drug candidate continue to

8. *Why is there a post-approval monitoring process?*

---

pharmacodynamic /fɑːməkəʊˈdaɪnæmɪk/ *adj*.	药效的
toxicity /tɒkˈsɪsəti/ *n*.	毒性；毒力
profile /ˈprəʊfaɪl/ *n*.	侧面；半面；轮廓
validate /ˈvælɪdeɪt/ *v*.	证实；确认；使有法律效力
regulatory /ˈregjələtəri/ *adj*.	监管的；具有监管权的；调整的
approval /əˈpruːvl/ *n*.	赞成；认可；通过
commercialization /kəˌmɜːʃəlaɪˈzeɪʃn/ *n*.	商业化；商品化
monitoring /ˈmɒnɪtərɪŋ/ *n*.	监控；监视；监督
grant /grænt/ *v/n*.	授予；允许；拨款

be monitored and evaluated. This includes adverse event reporting, **periodic** safety updates, and efficacy data collection.

The drug research and development process is complex and costly due to the need for extensive research, preclinical testing, clinical trials, and regulatory approvals. It typically requires years of work by highly skilled scientific researchers and costs millions of dollars to bring a single drug to market.

9. Why is the drug research and development process said to be complex and costly?

3.2 Key Technologies and Tools in Drug Development

Drug development is a complex and highly specialized process that involves multiple stages, from the initial discovery of a potential therapeutic agent to the final approval and marketing of a drug product. To support this process, a range of technologies and tools are commonly used to improve research, testing, and manufacturing efforts.

1. What supports a complex and highly specialized process of drug development?

One important aspect of drug development is the use of high-throughput screening (HTS) techniques. HTS allows researchers to test large libraries of compounds rapidly and efficiently, identifying those with the most promise as therapeutic agents. HTS typically involves **robotic** systems that **automate** the process of

2. What is the use of HTS techniques?

---

periodic /ˌpɪrɪˈɒdɪk/ *adj.*   定期的;周期的;间发性的
robotic /rəʊˈbɒtɪk/ *adj.*   机器人的;自动的
automate /ˈɔːtəmeɪt/ *v.*   使自动化

dispensing compounds, measuring their effects on cells or biochemical **assays**, and collecting data.

Computational tools are also essential in drug development, particularly in structure-based drug design. These tools allow researchers to model the three-dimensional structure of proteins and other **macromolecules**, predicting how potential drugs may bind to them and affect their function. Structure-based drug design is particularly valuable for attacking complex diseases like cancer, HIV/AIDS, and **neurodegenerative** disorders.

3. Why are computational tools essential in drug development?

Artificial intelligence (AI) and machine learning have also been applied increasingly to drug development. These technologies can help identify patterns in large **datasets**, predicting outcomes in clinical trials or optimizing the manufacturing process. AI **algorithms** can also be used to analyze scientific **literature** and other information sources, identifying novel therapeutic targets or synthetic routes for drugs.

4. What are the advantages of using AI in drug development?

In addition to these modern technologies, traditional methods like **organic** synthesis and **biochemistry** continue to play important roles in drug development.

5. Why are some traditional methods still used in drug

---

dispense /dɪˈspens/ *v*.　　　　　　分配;分发;配(药)
assay /ˈæsˌe/ *n*.　　　　　　　　检验;化验;分析
computational /ˌkɒmpjʊˈteɪʃənl/ *adj*.　计算的;计算机的
macromolecule /ˌmækrəˈmɒləˌkjʊl/ *n*.　高分子;巨大分子
neurodegenerative /ˌnjʊrəʊdɪˈdʒenərətɪv/ *adj*.　神经组织退化的
dataset /ˈdeɪtəset/ *n*.　　　　　　数据集
algorithm /ˈælgəˌrɪðəm/ *n*.　　　　算法;运算法则
literature /ˈlɪtrətʃər/ *n*.　　　　著述;文献;文学;文学作品
organic /ɔːrˈɡænɪk/ *adj*.　　　　　有机的;自然的;器官的
biochemistry /ˌbaɪəʊˈkemɪstrɪ/ *n*.　生物化学;生物化学过程

Organic synthesis is used to prepare structurally diverse compounds with the desired pharmacological properties, while biochemistry is essential for understanding the mechanisms of drug action and resistance at the **cellular** level.

development?

Finally, animal testing is an important **component** of drug development, particularly for compounds that may have toxic or other harmful effects in humans. Animal testing can help evaluate the safety and efficacy of drugs before clinical trials in humans begin, although there are **ethical concerns** associated with this practice.

6. What is the use of animal testing in drug development?

Overall, drug development involves a combination of modern and traditional technologies and tools, each playing a crucial role in the process of developing safe and effective drugs to treat human diseases.

Language Practice

I. Vocabulary Work

Complete each of the following sentences with a suitable word or expression given below.

target	synthetic	regulatory	organic
identification	candidate	approval	biochemistry
screening	potency	grant	cellular
evaluate	toxicity	periodic	concern
profile	validate	automate	dispense

---

cellular /ˈseljələr/ *adj*.　　　　　细胞的；由细胞组成的；蜂窝状的
component /kəmˈpəʊnənt/ *n*.　　　组成部分；成分
ethical /ˈeθɪkl/ *adj*.　　　　　　　伦理的；道德的
concern /kənˈsɜːrn/ *n*.　　　　　　担心；令人担心的事；关心

1. We need to _____ the effectiveness of this new drug candidate in a clinical trial before moving forward with its development.

2. The main concern during drug development is the potential _____ of the compound.

3. The FDA _____ process can take several years for a new drug to be approved.

4. Identifying the right _____ is crucial for the development of effective drugs.

5. There are _____ about the side effects of the new drug candidate.

6. The _____ drugs can be produced in a controlled environment, ensuring consistent quality and safety.

7. The _____ requirements for bringing a new drug to market are very strict and time-consuming.

8. The pharmacy must _____ the correct dosage of the medication to each patient.

9. The research team plans to conduct _____ evaluations of the drug's efficacy in patients.

10. The preclinical studies are designed to _____ the safety and efficacy of the new drug candidate.

11. The toxicology _____ of the drug candidate showed no concerning side effects in animal models.

12. _____ of side effects is essential for ensuring the safety of new drugs.

13. The foundation has _____ funding to several promising drug development projects in the early stages.

14. The FDA requires that all drugs go through a rigorous _____ process before approval.

15. The research team is exploring the use of natural _____ compounds as potential sources of new drugs.

II. Word Building

Study the Prefixes, Suffixes and Roots in the following grid, and then provide the corresponding word based on the given definition.

Prefixes	Meaning	Example
peri-	"around" or "close to"（围绕；接近）	periodic
robo-	"relating to a robot"（与机器人有关的）	robotic
Suffixes		
-ation	"the action or process of doing something"（动作或过程）	identification
-al	"the act or state of"（行为或状态）	approval
Roots		
bio	"life"（生命）	biochemistry
merch	"commerce" or "trading"（商业；贸易）	commercialize
val	"value" or "worth"（价值）	evaluation
cell	"the basic unit of life"（细胞；生命基本单位）	cellular

1. relating to cells _____

2. the study of living organisms _____

3. the study of the chemical processes in living organisms _____

4. extremely valuable, beyond measure _____

5. relating to the buying and selling of goods _____

6. to turn something into a commercial venture _____

7. situated near or surrounding something, especially in relation to it _____

8. the field of technology concerned with the design, construction, and control of robots _____

9. the act of changing or adapting something to make it different _____

10. the act of arriving at a place _____

III. Structure & Function

Present participles（现在分词）can function as adjectives describing or modifying a noun or a pronoun in a sentence. Present participle phrases can also be used as adverbials to indicate the time, cause, result or accompanying condition of the situation. For example:

The process of drug research and development is complex and costly, typically taking 10~15 years and millions of dollars to bring a new drug to market.

（现在分词短语作为方式状语，描述药物研究和开发的过程通常是如何进行的，即通常需要 10～15 年时间和数百万美元才能将新药推向市场。）

HTS typically involves robotic systems that automate the process of dispensing compounds , measuring their effects on cells or biochemical assays , and collecting data . （两个现在分词短语在句中做伴随状语，说明机器人系统在 HTS 中执行的具体任务。）

These technologies can help identify patterns in large datasets , predicting outcomes in clinical trials or optimizing the manufacturing process . （现在分词短语作为结果状语，说明这些技术能够预测临床试验的结果或优化生产过程）

Drug development involves a combination of modern and traditional technologies and tools , each playing a crucial role in the process of developing safe and effective drugs to treat human diseases . （现在分词短语用于独立结构，作为方式状语描述现代和传统技术与工具在药物开发过程中各自扮演的关键角色。）

The present participle phrases are widely used in English for medical purposes, which can accurately describe actions, states, and relationships, making the expression of medical English clearer and more accurate.

Translate the following sentences into English , using in each a present participle phrase .

1. 在经过必要的准备工作后，我们现在可以开始进行这个项目了。

_____

_____

2. 在分析临床试验数据时，科学家们发现了一种之前未被注意到的潜在副作用。

_____

_____

3. 尽管遇到了许多障碍，研究团队仍然坚持不懈，最终在医学领域取得了突破性的发现。

_____

_____

4. 经过多年的专注研究，我们成功开发出一种新药，在治疗这种疾病方面取得了重大进展。

_____

_____

5. 由于研究人员采取的创新方法，一种之前无法治愈的疾病现在可以得到治疗，进一步证实了他们的假设。

_____

_____

IV. Audio-visual Exercise

A. Sentence Dictation

Please listen to each sentence twice. First listening is for you to understand the general meaning of the sentence. Try to repeat the sentence after you listen to it for a second time，and then write down the whole sentence during the pauses. You'll listen to all the sentences for a third time for checking your dictation.

1. Advances in technology _____

_____

2. Computational methods _____

_____

3. Artificial organs _____

_____

4. Bioprinting _____

_____

5. In-vitro cell culture systems _____

_____

B. Visual Comprehension

Watch a video three times and decide whether each of the following statements is true（T）or false（F）.

_____ 1. You need to know basically there are three main clinical phases and trials that have to go on to develop a vaccine.

_____ 2. Phase I evaluates safety and efficacy of a vaccine across various populations.

_____ 3. You have to know that the process of developing any vaccine normally takes decades of time.

_____ 4. "12 to 18 months" is absolutely the minimum time period that would take to develop a vaccine.

_____ 5. The work that had been done on SARS helped cut certain steps for development of COVID-19 vaccine.

_____ 6. We know that we need to get a different vaccine for COVID-19 one every year, like we do for influenza.

_____ 7. We know that being infected with COVID-19 doesn't give you long-term immunity.

V. Extended Reading

Read the following dialogue between Dr. Pharmed and students about the basic process of drug research and development, and complete the dialogue with a suitable phrase or sentence from the grid.

Dr. Pharmed: Good morning, everybody. Today, we will be discussing the basic process of drug research and development.

Student 1: Thank you, Dr. Pharmed. We are eager to learn about this important topic.

Dr. Pharmed: The basic process of drug research and development involves several stages, including discovery, pre-clinical studies, clinical trials, regulatory approval, and commercialization. In the discovery stage, __1__ that may be effective in treating those targets. These compounds are then tested in pre-clinical studies to evaluate their safety and efficacy. If a compound shows promise, it moves on to clinical trials, where it is tested on human participants to assess its effectiveness and safety. Once clinical trials are complete and the data is reviewed by regulatory agencies, drugs can receive approval for use in patients. Finally, once drugs have been approved for use, __2__, which includes manufacturing, distributing, and marketing the drug to patients.

Student 2: Can you explain the role of pharmacologists in drug research and development?

Dr. Pharmed: Absolutely. As pharmacologists, our role in drug research and development is multifaceted. We conduct research to identify new drug targets and develop new compounds that may be effective in treating various diseases. We also conduct clinical trials to evaluate the safety and efficacy of these compounds in humans. Additionally, __3__ to ensure that drug development is conducted in an ethical and responsible manner. Our expertise in pharmacokinetics, pharmacodynamics, and toxicology is also critical for ensuring that drugs are developed and manufactured safely and effectively.

Student 3: What challenges do drug researchers face during the development process?

Dr. Pharmed: There are many challenges that drug researchers face during the development process. One major challenge is the high cost of drug development, as __4__ . Another challenge is the time it takes to bring drugs to market, as the process can take several years or even decades. Additionally, there are legal and regulatory challenges that must be overcome in order to bring drugs to market, such as obtaining approval from regulatory agencies and ensuring compliance with international trade agreements. Despite these challenges, __5__ that improve patient outcomes and advance our understanding of disease prevention and management.

Student 4: Thank you for sharing this information with us, professor. We feel much more prepared to discuss drug research and development with our future patients.

Dr. Pharmed: You're welcome. Remember, __6__ that relies on the expertise of many different professionals. By staying informed and engaged in this field, we can help ensure that patients around the world have access to safe and effective treatments for a wide range of diseases.

_____	1	A. they move through the commercialization process
_____	2	B. drug research and development is a complex and ongoing process
_____	3	C. researchers identify potential drug targets and develop compounds
_____	4	D. drug researchers continue to work tirelessly to develop new treatments
_____	5	
_____	6	E. It ensures that patients have access to safe and effective treatments
		F. we collaborate with other researchers and healthcare professionals
		G. it requires extensive research and testing before drugs can be brought to market
		H. we conduct research to identify new drug targets and develop new compounds

VI. Topics for Discussion and Essay-writing

1. Why is drug development a complex and highly specialized process?

2. What are the main objectives of the three phases of a drug clinical trial?

3. Why is artificial intelligence (AI) being applied increasingly to drug development?

Chapter IV

Clinical Application of Drugs

4.1　Issues Involved in Drug Clinical Application

Clinical application of drugs involves several issues that need to be considered for safe and effective treatment. Some of the key issues are:

Drug efficacy: The drug's ability to achieve its intended therapeutic effect in the target patient population is an important consideration. It is essential to **conduct** clinical trials to assess the drug's efficacy and safety before recommending it for use in patients.

1. How to assess the drug's efficacy and safety?

Drug toxicity: The potential side effects of a drug should be carefully evaluated during its development and clinical trial phases. Even when a drug has been approved by regulatory agencies, it may still cause adverse effects in some patients. Therefore, monitoring of drug toxicity is crucial for ensuring patient safety.

2. Why is monitoring of drug toxicity crucial for ensuring patient safety?

Drug interactions: Drugs can interact with other medications, herbal supplements, or foods, potentially

---

conduct /kənˈdʌkt/ v.　　　　　　　进行;组织;实施

leading to adverse effects or reduced efficacy. It is essential to consider drug interactions when prescribing or administering drugs to ensure that patients receive **optimal** care.

3. What are the poten-tial risks of drug interactions?

Drug dosage: The appropriate dosage of a drug is critical for achieving desired therapeutic effects while minimizing the risk of side effects. Healthcare professionals must determine the **appropriate** dosage based on the patient's age, weight, medical history, and other factors.

4. What factors are considered when determining the appropri-ate drug dosage for a patient?

Drug **formulations**: The form in which a drug is delivered (e. g., tablets, capsules, injections) can affect its **bioavailability** and pharmacokinetics. It is essential to consider these aspects when selecting the appropriate drug formulation for a particular patient.

5. What affect the bioavail-ability and pharmacokinetics of drugs?

Drug resistance: Drug resistance refers to the ability of bacteria, viruses, or other **pathogens** to develop resist-ance to a particular drug over time. As a result, health-care professionals must monitor the emergence of drug resistance and adjust their treatment plans accordingly.

6. What is drug resis-tance?

Economic considerations: The cost of developing, manufacturing, and distributing drugs can vary significantly depending on factors such as market demand, patent protection, and regulatory requirements. Healthcare professionals must balance the benefits of using a specific drug against its costs to ensure that patients receive **affordable** treatment options.

7. What factors impact the cost of drug development, manufacturing, and distribu-tion?

---

optimal /ˈɒptɪməl/ *adj*.　　　　　最优的；最佳的；最适的
appropriate /əˈprəʊprɪət/ *adj*.　　适当的；合适的；恰当的
formulation /ˌfɔːmjəˈleʃən/ *n*.　　（药品或化妆品的）配方；配方产品
bioavailability /ˌbaɪəʊrˌveɪləˈbɪlɪt/ *n*.　　生物药效率；生物利用度
pathogen /ˈpæθədʒən/ *n*.　　　　病原体
affordable /əˈfɔːrdəbl/ *adj*.　　　价格合理的；多数人买得起的

4.2　Drug Indications

Drug indications refer to the conditions or diseases for which a specific medication is prescribed or recommended. These **indications** are based on clinical research, pharmacological properties, and toxicity profiles of the drug. Indications help healthcare professionals choose appropriate medications for their patients and ensure that they receive the best possible treatment.

1. How do drug indications help healthcare professionals?

For example, if a patient has a bacterial infection, an antibiotic may be prescribed as the drug of choice due to its **antimicrobial** properties. Similarly, if a patient has high blood pressure, a medication like an **angiotensin**-converting enzyme (ACE) inhibitor may be prescribed to lower blood pressure levels.

2. What are some examples of drug indications that healthcare professionals commonly encounter in their practice?

Indications can also vary depending on the patient's age, medical history, and other factors. Healthcare professionals consider all these factors when prescribing drugs to ensure that the treatment is safe and effective for the patient.

3. What factors should healthcare professionals consider when prescribing drugs to patients?

Drug indications are typically listed on the drug's label and provide important information for healthcare providers about when and how the drug should be used.

4. What is the purpose of drug indications?

---

indication /ˌɪndɪˈkeɪʃn/ n.　　　适应证;表明;标示
antimicrobial /ˌæntɪmaɪˈkrəʊbɪrl/ adj.　抗菌的
angiotensin /ˌændʒɪəʊˈtensən/ n.　　血管紧缩素

4.3   Drug Adverse Reactions

Drug adverse reactions (ADRs) refer to any harmful or unpleasant medical events that occur in patients as a result of using drugs. These reactions may range from mild skin **rashes** or headaches to life-threatening conditions such as liver failure or **renal** failure.

ADRs can be classified into different types depending on their causes and characteristics. The most common types include hypersensitivity reactions, **idiosyncratic** reactions, dose-related reactions, and adverse drug interactions. Hypersensitivity reactions occur in patients who are sensitive to a drug or its metabolites, causing allergic reactions such as skin rashes or **respiratory** symptoms. Idiosyncratic reactions are **unique** to certain individuals and are not related to the dose of the drug, often with serious consequences. Dose-related reactions occur when the dose of the drug is **exceeded**, causing poisoning symptoms or other harmful effects. Adverse drug interactions occur when two or more drugs interact with each other to **enhance** their pharmacological effects or create new adverse reactions.

1. What are the potential consequences of drug adverse reactions for patients?

2. What are the most common types of drug adverse reactions and how are they classified?

---

rash /ræʃ/ *n*.　　　　　　　疹子;皮疹
renal /ˈriːnəl/ *adj*.　　　　　肾脏的;肾的
idiosyncratic /ˌɪdɪəsɪŋˈkrætɪk/ *adj*.　特异应性的;特异体质的;乖僻的
respiratory /ˈrespərətɔːrɪ/ *adj*.　呼吸的
unique /juˈniːk/ *adj*.　　　　独有的;特有的
exceed /ɪkˈsiːd/ *v*.　　　　　(数量)超过;超越(限制、规定)
enhance /ɪnˈhæns/ *v*.　　　　增强;提高;增加

ADRs can also vary depending on the type of drug used. For example, **antitumor** drugs are associated with serious **myelosuppression** and **immunosuppression**, affecting patients' white blood cell count and immune function, increasing the risk of infection and other serious consequences. **Antihypertensive** drugs may cause **hypotension**, **bradycardia**, and other **cardiovascular** reactions. Antibiotic drugs may cause allergic reactions, liver damage, and other side effects.

To **minimize** the **occurrence** of ADRs, doctors need to choose appropriate drugs according to patients' conditions and adjust the dosage based on individual differences. In addition, patients should actively cooperate with doctors during treatment and report any **discomfort** they experience **promptly** to ensure that their safety is effectively protected.

3. *What are some common side effects of antitumor drugs, antihypertensive drugs, and antibiotic drugs?*

4. *What role do patients play in minimizing the risk of drug adverse reactions?*

---

antitumor /ˌæntɪˈtjʊmər/ *adj*.　　　　抗肿瘤的；抗癌的

myelosuppression /ˈmaɪləʊsʌpreʃn/ *n*.　骨髓抑制

immunosuppression /ˌɪmjʊnəʊsəˈpreʃn/ *n*.　免疫抑制

antihypertensive /ˌæntɪhaɪpərˈtensɪve/ *adj*.　抗高血压的

hypotension /ˌhaɪpəˈtenʃən/ *n*.　　　　低血压

bradycardia /ˌbrædɪˈkɑːdɪə/ *n*.　　　　心动过缓

cardiovascular /ˌkɑːdɪəʊˈvæskjələ(r)/ *adj*.　心血管的

minimize /ˈmɪnɪmaɪz/ *v*.　　　　　　使减至最低程度；使保持最低程度

occurrence /əˈkɜːrəns/ *n*.　　　　　　发生；出现

discomfort /dɪsˈkʌmfərt/ *n*.　　　　　不舒服；不适

promptly /ˈprɒmptlɪ/ *adv*.　　　　　　立即；迅速地；及时

4.4 Precautions for Medication

When taking medication, it is important to take certain **precautions** to ensure that you receive the best possible care and avoid potential side effects or complications. Here are some general precautions to be taken when taking medication:

Read the label carefully: Be sure to read the medication label carefully before taking any medication, paying close attention to the instructions for dosing, administration, and any special precautions or warnings.

Follow the prescribed dosage: Always follow the prescribed dosage of your medication, even if you feel better or think you can skip a dose. Overdosing can lead to serious side effects or complications.

Tell your healthcare provider about all medications: Be sure to tell your healthcare provider about all medications, including **over-the-counter** drugs, supplements, and herbal remedies, as well as any allergies or medical conditions you may have.

Avoid alcohol and tobacco: Avoid drinking alcohol and smoking tobacco while taking certain medications, as these can interact with the medication and increase the risk of side effects or complications.

Report any adverse reactions: If you experience any adverse reactions or side effects while taking your medication, be sure to report them to your healthcare

1. What precautions should be paid attention to when taking medicine?

2. What information should patients be aware of about medication label?

3. What information should you tell your healthcare provider about?

4. How can alcohol and tobacco affect the effectiveness of certain medications?

5. What should you do if you experience adverse reactions

---

precaution /prɪˈkɔːʃn/ n. 预防措施;防备

over-the-counter /ˌəʊvər ðə ˈkaʊntər/ adj. 无需处方可买到的;非处方的

provider immediately.

Keep track of refills: Make sure you keep track of when your medication refills are due and arrange for them in advance if necessary, to avoid running out of medication.

Store medications properly: Be sure to store your medications properly, following the instructions on the label or provided by your healthcare provider. Some medications should be stored in a cool, dry place, while others should be kept in the refrigerator.

or side effects while taking your medication?

6. How should you store your medications properly?

Language Practice

I. Vocabulary Work

Complete each of the following sentences with a suitable word or expression given below.

conduct	respiratory	hypotension	cardiovascular
optimal	unique	precaution	minimize
appropriate	exceed	keep track of	occurrence
formulation	enhance	refill	discomfort
antimicrobial	indication	pathogen	promptly

1. Proper _____ of experiments is crucial in pharmaceutical research to obtain accurate and reliable data.

2. One of the challenges in drug development is identifying new _____ for drugs that have already been approved, as this requires additional clinical trials and regulatory approval.

3. Pharmaceutical companies conduct clinical trials to evaluate the effects of their drugs on blood pressure, including the potential to cause _____.

keep track of 跟踪;记录
refill /rɪˈfɪl/ *n*. 重新配药

4. The goal of pharmaceutical development is to _____ the efficacy of drugs while minimizing side effects.

5. In the preclinical testing phase, researchers seek to determine the _____ dosing schedule for the new drug candidate.

6. Each new drug candidate brings _____ challenges and opportunities during the pharmaceutical development process.

7. Pharmaceutical companies invest significant resources into developing new _____ that improve the stability, solubility, and bioavailability of drugs, ultimately enhancing their efficacy and safety.

8. Regulatory agencies require that pharmaceutical companies take necessary _____ to ensure the quality and efficacy of their products, including implementing stringent manufacturing processes and quality control measures.

9. The new drug candidate _____ expectations in preclinical trials, demonstrating a significant improvement in efficacy over existing treatments.

10. The _____ of side effects is closely monitored during clinical trials to assess the safety profile of new drugs.

11. The development of new drugs aims to minimize patient _____ and improve quality of life.

12. During the clinical trial process, it is essential to _____ patient progress and any adverse events that occur.

13. By offering _____ options, the pharmacy can provide patients with a convenient and cost-effective way to manage their medication.

14. The _____ drug is being developed with the aim of reducing the spread of infectious diseases and improving patient outcomes.

15. The _____ health of patients is a key consideration in the development of new drugs, ensuring their safety and efficacy.

II. Word Building

Study the Prefixes, Suffixes and Roots in the following grid, and then provide the corresponding word based on the given definition.

Prefixes	Meaning	Example
re-	"again"（重新）	refill
mini-	"smallest or least"（最小的）	minimize
Suffixes		
-ory	indicating a relationship or connection（表明关系或联系的形容词后缀）	respiratory
-ly	added to the adjective to form the adverb（副词后缀）	promptly
Roots		
path(o)	"suffering" or "disease"（病；疾病）	pathogen
micro	"small"（微小）	antimicrobial
respire	"breathe"（呼吸）	respiratory
cardio	"heart"（心；心脏）	cardiovascular

1. to construct something again, typically after it has been damaged or destroyed

　　——————

2. relating to the process of breathing, specifically involving the organs and structures involved in respiration

　　——————

3. to reduce the amount of something that is present or existing 　——————

4. the study of diseases of the heart and the cardiovascular system 　——————

5. occurs at a regular interval or frequency 　——————

6. related to or involving the giving of advice or guidance 　——————

7. the study of the causes, processes, and effects of diseases, typically in the context of medical science

　　——————

8. a very small organism, especially one that is not visible to the naked eye

　　——————

9. quickly and without delay 　——————

10. of or relating to the heart and blood vessels 　——————

III. Structure & Function

　　Modal verbs（情态动词）in English express various meanings such as ability, possibility, necessity, advice, prediction, and willingness. For example：

　　Drugs <u>can</u> interact with other medications, herbal supplements, or foods, *potentially leading to adverse effects or reduced efficacy*. ("can" expresses ability or possibility)

Even when a drug has been approved by regulatory agencies, it may still cause adverse effects in some patients. ("may" expresses possibility or probability)

Some medications should be stored in a cool, dry place, while others should be kept in the refrigerator. ("should" expresses necessity)

Healthcare professionals must balance the benefits of using a specific drug against its costs to ensure that patients receive affordable treatment options. ("must" expresses necessity)

Here are more examples of how these modal verbs are used in science and medical literature:

1. Ability:

The new drug can effectively treat cancer.

2. Possibility:

The experiment may produce unexpected results.

3. Necessity:

Healthcare professionals must determine the appropriate dosage based on the patient's age, weight, medical history, and other factors.

The potential side effects of a drug should be carefully evaluated during its development and clinical trial phases.

4. Advice:

Patients should actively cooperate with doctors during treatment and report any discomfort they experience promptly to ensure that their safety is effectively protected.

5. Prediction:

The vaccine will be available to the public by next year.

6. Willingness:

I would like to volunteer at the local hospital.

Modal verbs can also be used to express our understanding, guesses or assumptions about past events, but they do not necessarily represent what actually happened. For example:

He must have finished his work last night，because his desk is clean．（must have done 这个结构表示对过去发生事情的强烈推测，但无法证实）

You should have called me when you knew you were going to be late．（should have done 这个结构表示对过去应该做某事却没有做的后悔或责备）

He can have finished his work，but I'm not sure．（can have done 这种结构表示一种较为不确定的可能性）

She could have come to the party，but she was probably busy．（could have done 这种结构表示一种较为可能的可能性）

He may have gone to the store already．（may have done 这个结构表示对过去可能发生的事情的推测）

If we had started earlier，we would have reached the destination before dark．（would have done 这个结构表示对过去可能发生的事情的虚拟，通常用于假设过去发生了什么，而实际上并没有发生）

Translate the following sentences into English，using in each a modal verb．

1. 患者在接受治疗后症状明显改善，因此这种药物肯定产生了积极的效果。

   _____

   _____

2. 如果医生开出了不同的药物，药物对患者健康的负面影响本可以最小化。

   _____

   _____

3. 试验结果不确定，所以研究人员本来应该进行更为严格的实验来确认药物的疗效。

   _____

   _____

4. 患者对药物的反应肯定不是由药物本身引起的，因为这是一种已知且经过测试的药物。

   _____

   _____

5. 如果试验包括了更多样的患者人群，这种药物本来会更有效，并且在特定群体中引起不良反应也会更小。

IV. Audio-visual Exercise

A. Sentence Dictation

Please listen to each sentence twice. First listening is for you to understand the general meaning of the sentence. Try to repeat the sentence after you listen to it for a second time, and then write down the whole sentence during the pauses. You'll listen to all the sentences for a third time for checking your dictation.

1. Clinical application of drugs _____

   _____

2. The potential side effects _____

   _____

3. Drug indications _____

   _____

4. Drug adverse reactions _____

   _____

5. Always follow _____

   _____

B. Visual Comprehension

Watch a video three times and decide whether each of the following statements is true（T）or false（F）.

_____ 1. The story affects potentially millions of Americans who take statin drugs.

_____ 2. New evidence suggests these drugs may be a risk factor for type 2 diabetes.

_____ 3. They followed more than 150,000 women over 50 with type 2 diabetes for about 10 years.

_____ 4. The study found that women taking statin drugs had a 48% greater chance of developing type 2 diabetes.

_____ 5. Doctors don't know that heart disease is one of the major complications of diabetes.

_____ 6. Judy Berg's case is a reminder that every drug has both risks and benefits.

_____ 7. The video clip is mainly about how statin drugs could cut the cholesterol level.

V. Extended Reading

Read the following dialogue between Dr. Pharmed and students about drug adverse reactions, and choose the best answer to each question according to the dialogue.

Dr. Pharmed: Good morning, everyone. Today, we'll be discussing drug adverse reactions. What do you think are some of the most common adverse reactions to medications?

Student 1: Well, I think that nausea and vomiting are pretty common. Some people can develop an allergic reaction to certain medications as well.

Dr. Pharmed: Yes, those are definitely some common ones. It's important to always inform your prescribing doctor if you experience any side effects while taking a medication, especially if they are severe or persistent.

Student 2: Can you give us an example of when it's important to report a side effect?

Dr. Pharmed: Sure. Let's say a patient is prescribed a medication for high blood pressure, but they start experiencing severe dizziness and lightheadedness. If this continues despite the patient's normal diet and activity level, it could be a sign of a serious side effect. In this case, it would be important for the patient to inform their healthcare provider so that the appropriate action can be taken.

Student 3: Are there any other factors that can affect drug interactions?

Dr. Pharmed: Yes, there are many factors that can affect drug interactions. For example, if a patient is taking multiple medications at once, each one may interact with the others in different ways. Additionally, certain foods, herbs, or supplements may interact with medications and increase or decrease their effectiveness. It's important for patients to disclose all the medications they are taking, including over-the-counter supplements, to their healthcare providers so that potential interactions can be identified and addressed.

Student 4: What about drug resistance? How does that affect drug therapy?

Dr. Pharmed: Drug resistance refers to the development of bacteria, viruses, or other pathogens that are resistant to a particular medication. This can lead to treatment failure and increase the risk of complications. To minimize the risk of drug resistance, it's important to follow proper medication use protocols, such as completing full courses of antibiotics even if symptoms improve early on. Additionally, maintaining good hygiene practices like handwashing can help prevent the spread of resistant bacteria.

Student 5: Thank you for your time today. We learned a lot about drug adverse reactions!

Dr. Pharmed: You're welcome! Remember, it's always important to communicate with your healthcare provider about any side effects you experience while taking medications. Your provider can help determine whether the side effects are related to the medication or another underlying condition and provide guidance on how to manage them effectively.

1. Which of the following is NOT a common adverse reaction to medications?
   A. Nausea.   B. Vomiting.
   C. Allergic reaction.   D. Severe dizziness.

2. Why is it important to report side effects to a healthcare provider?
   A. To ensure the patient is taking the correct dosage of the medication.
   B. To identify potential drug interactions or other serious side effects.
   C. To determine if the medication is causing any long-term damage.
   D. To ensure the patient is following the doctor's advice on lifestyle changes.

3. Which of the following factors can affect drug interactions?
   A. The patient's age.

    B. The patient's gender.

    C. The patient's genetic makeup.

    D. The type of medication being taken.

4. What is the best advice for patients to avoid potential drug interactions?

    A. Disclose all the medications they are taking to their healthcare providers.

    B. Avoid taking any supplements or herbal remedies with their medication.

    C. Only take medication prescribed by their primary care provider.

    D. Always take their medication on an empty stomach.

5. Why is it important to complete full courses of antibiotics even if symptoms improve early on?

    A. To ensure that the bacteria are completely eliminated from the body.

    B. To reduce the risk of spreading resistant bacteria to others.

    C. To prevent the development of drug resistance.

    D. To save money on future medical expense.

VI. Topics for Discussion and Essay-writing

1. Why should a drug approved by the regulatory authorities be still monitored for its toxicity?

2. Which is more important: to weigh the efficacy of a drug or the patient's financial burden when prescribing drugs?

3. What should patients pay attention to when taking their medication to ensure the best efficacy while avoiding possible side effects?

Chapter V

Legal and Ethical Issues Concerning Drugs

5.1 Drug Naming

The International **Nonproprietary** Name (INN) is a standardized name for drugs that is used worldwide to identify and **distinguish** different pharmaceutical products. The INN is assigned by the World Health Organization (WHO) and is used in place of the **brand-name** drug to refer to the same product. This allows generic drugs, which are produced by different companies under **license** from the original manufacturer, to be more easily **interchangeable** with **branded** drugs in various countries.

A drug's "**generic name**," "patent name," or

1. What is the purpose of the International Nonproprietary Name (INN)?

2. Who assigns the INN?

---

nonproprietary /ˌnɒnprəˈpraɪɪˌterɪ/ *adj.*		非专有的
distinguish /dɪˈstɪŋgwɪʃ/ *v.*		区分;使有别于
brand-name /ˈbrændˌneɪm/ *n.*		品牌名
license /ˈlaɪsns/ *n.*		许可证;特许
interchangeable /ˌɪntərˈtʃeɪndʒəbl/ *adj.*		可交换的;可交替的
branded /ˈbrændɪd/ *adj.*		有品牌的;打有烙印的
generic name /dʒəˈnerɪk neɪm/ *n.*		通用名;总名称;属名

"brand-name" refers to the specific product name assigned by the manufacturer of the drug.

The generic name is the nonproprietary name used by pharmaceutical companies to refer to their products. It is typically composed of five parts: the active **ingredient**, the chemical structure, the country of origin, the therapeutic use, and the year of approval. For example, the generic name for a drug called **metformin** may be 500 mg metformin extended-release for oral administration, US, **antihyperglycemic**.

The patent name is the **proprietary** name used by the **manufacturer** to protect their **intellectual** property rights. It is usually different from the generic name and is not publicly available.

The brand-name is the specific product name that is marketed and sold by the manufacturer. It is designed to be **memorable** and **attractive** to **consumers** and can include various marketing elements such as **logos**, **slogans**, and packaging. The brand-name is protected by **trademark** laws and cannot be used by other

3. How does the generic name differ from the brand-name and patent name?

4. What are the components typically included in a drug's generic name?

5. Why is the brand-name protected by trademark laws?

6. What is the purpose of designing a brand-name?

---

ingredient /ɪnˈɡriːdɪənt/ n.　　　　　　组成部分;(烹调的)原料
metformin /metˈfɔːmɪn/ n.　　　　　　　二甲双胍(抗糖尿病药、降血糖药)
antihyperglycemic /ˌæntɪhaɪpəɡlɪˈsemɪk/ adj.　　抗高血糖药
proprietary /prəˈpraɪəterɪ/ adj.　　　　专有的;专利的
manufacturer /ˌmænjʊˈfæktʃərər/ n.　　制造商;制造厂
intellectual /ˌɪntəˈlektʃʊəl/ adj.　　　　智力的;有才智的;需用智力的
memorable /ˈmemərəbl/ adj.　　　　　　难忘的;值得纪念的;显著的
attractive /əˈtræktɪv/ adj.　　　　　　　吸引人的;有魅力的;好看的
consumer /kənˈsuːmər/ n.　　　　　　　消费者;顾客
logo /ˈləʊɡəʊ/ n.　　　　　　　　　　　标识;标志;徽标
slogan /ˈsləʊɡən/ n.　　　　　　　　　　短语;标语;口号
trademark /ˈtreɪdmɑːrk/ n.　　　　　　　(注册)商标

manufacturers without **permission**.

A new drug is named after the **sponsoring** company, which is typically a pharmaceutical company that invests in the research and development of a new drug. There are several principles for naming a new drug, including:

The name should be **descriptive** and easy to understand.

The name should not be **misleading** or **confusing**.

The name should not be too long or complicated.

The name should be unique and not already in use by another company or product.

The name should be appropriate for the target population and the intended use of the drug.

The name should reflect the safety and efficacy of the drug.

The name should be **consistent** with existing drug names and **terminology**.

The name should be culturally **sensitive** and appropriate for different countries and regions.

According to the regulations, if there are no INN names in traditional Chinese medicine and biological drugs, they can be treated as appropriate, while chemical drugs should be named according to their active

7. How are new drugs named, and what are the principles guiding the naming process?

permission /pərˈmɪʃn/ n.　准许；许可证
sponsoring /ˈspɒnsərɪŋ/ adj.　赞助的；资助的
descriptive /dɪˈskrɪptɪv/ adj.　描写的；叙述的
misleading /mɪsˈliːdɪŋ/ adj.　误导性的；骗人的；引入歧途的
confusing /kənˈfjuːzɪŋ/ adj.　难以理解的
consistent /kənˈsɪstənt/ adj.　一致的；连贯的；始终如一的
terminology /ˌtɜːrmɪˈnɒlədʒɪ/ n.　术语；专门名词；术语学
sensitive /ˈsensətɪv/ adj.　敏感的；过敏的；灵敏的

ingredients. The World Health Organization requires an INN only for trade names approved in at least two countries worldwide. Moreover, an INN cannot be the same as an existing INN, and must be able to **pronounce** accurately, clearly and write correctly.

8. What are the requirements for an INN according to the World Health Organization?

5.2 Drug Registration Procedures

Drug **registration procedures** refer to the process of obtaining approval and registration for a drug in a given country. This involves conducting preclinical studies, conducting clinical trials, obtaining approval from regulatory authorities, **registering** the drug, and **undergoing** post-marketing **surveillance**. The goal of these procedures is to ensure that drugs are safe and effective before they are made available to the public. Drug registration procedures vary between countries, but they typically involve similar steps.

1. What are drug registration procedures aimed at?

Drug registration procedures consist of the following steps:

Preclinical studies: Before a drug can be registered, it must undergo preclinical studies to evaluate its safety and efficacy in animal models.

2. How many steps do drug registration procedures consist of?

Clinical trials: After preclinical studies, the drug

3. Which procedure is a must

---

pronounce /prəˈnaʊns/ v.　　　　发……的音；宣称；宣布
registration /ˌredʒɪˈstreɪʃn/ n.　　注册；登记；挂号
procedure /prəˈsiːdʒər/ n.　　　　程序；步骤
register /ˈredʒɪstər/ v.　　　　　给……注册；登记
undergo /ˌʌndərˈɡoʊ/ v.　　　　经历；忍受
surveillance /sɜːrˈveɪləns/ n.　　监督；管制

must undergo clinical trials in human subjects to confirm its safety and effectiveness.

in order to confirm a drug's safety and effectiveness in human subjects?

Approval from the Drug Administration: The drug must be approved by the Drug Administration before it can be marketed in China.

Registration: Once the drug has been approved, it must be registered with the Drug Administration to obtain a registration **certificate**.

Listing on the National Medical Products Information System (NMPA): The drug must also be listed on the NMPA to ensure that patients have access to accurate and up-to-date information about the drug.

4. Where can you get the latest information about a drug?

Post-marketing surveillance: After the drug is registered and listed on the NMPA, it must undergo post-marketing surveillance to monitor its safety and effectiveness over time.

5.3   Drug Advertisements

The **legal requirements** for **advertising** drugs vary by country and **jurisdiction**. However, in general, drug advertisements must **adhere to** strict regulations and guidelines to ensure the safety and effectiveness of the products being advertised.

1. What is required for a pharmaceutical company when advertising its products?

---

certificate /sə'tɪfɪkət/ *n.*   证明；证书
post-marketing   上市后
legal /'liːgl/ *adj.*   合法的
requirement /rɪ'kwaɪərmənt/ *n.*   要求；必要条件
advertise /'ædvərtaɪz/ *v.*   宣传；做广告
jurisdiction /ˌdʒʊrɪs'dɪkʃn/ *n.* 司法权；管辖权
adhere to   遵循；坚持

In many countries, including the United States, drug advertisements must include information about the potential risks and side effects of the product, as well as any contraindications or warnings. Additionally, advertisements may **be subject to** clinical trial results, which must be made available to the public through a **registry** or **database**.

Furthermore, drug manufacturers are required to **disclose** certain information about their products, such as the ingredients, dosage instructions, and intended use. They must also **comply with labeling** requirements, including providing clear and accurate information about the product's intended use and any potential side effects or interactions with other medications or treatments.

Advertising a drug that does not **conform to** legal regulations can have serious consequences, including:

Legal action: Advertising a drug without proper approval or **authorization** from regulatory authorities can result in **lawsuits** and **fines**.

Public safety: Advertising a drug that is not safe for **consumption** can put the public at risk of harm.

2. What is the essential element of a drug advertisement?

3. What does a law-breaking advertisement for a drug contribute to?

---

be subject to	受支配;从属于
registry /ˈredʒɪstrɪ/ *n.*	登记处
database /ˈdeɪtəbeɪs/ *n.*	数据库
disclose /dɪsˈkləʊz/ *v.*	揭露;使公开
comply with	服从;遵守
labeling /ˈleɪblɪŋ/ *n.*	标贴;标志
conform to	符合;遵照
authorization /ˌɔːθərəˈzeɪʃn/ *n.*	批准;授权(书)
lawsuit /ˈlɔːsuːt/ *n.*	诉讼;诉讼案件
fine /faɪn/ *n.*	罚款
consumption /kənˈsʌmpʃn/ *n.*	消费;消耗量

Reputation damage: Advertising a drug that does not meet legal standards can damage the **reputation** of the manufacturer and the brand.

Legal **liability**: The manufacturer may be held **liable** for any harm caused by their drug if it is found to be unsafe or **ineffective**.

Financial loss: Legal **penalties** and fines can result in significant financial losses for the manufacturer.

4. Why are the legal requirements for advertising drugs necessary?

Overall, the legal requirements for advertising drugs are designed to protect consumers from false or misleading information and ensure that they have access to accurate and up-to-date information about the products they are considering using.

Language Practice

I. Vocabulary Work

Complete each of the following sentences with a suitable word or expression given below.

distinguish	proprietary	misleading	adhere to
license	intellectual	consistent	be subject to
ingredient	memorable	registration	comply with
penalty	sensitive	surveillance	conform to
permission	trademark	consumption	liability

1. The drug's label clearly states its _____ and their respective concentrations.

---

reputation /ˌrepjʊˈteɪʃn/ *n.*   名誉；名声
liability /ˌlaɪəˈbɪlətɪ/ *n.*   责任；倾向；债务
liable /ˈlaɪəbl/ *adj.*   有责任的；有义务的
ineffective /ˌɪnɪˈfektɪv/ *adj.*   无效果的；无效率的
penalty /ˈpenəltɪ/ *n.*   惩罚；刑罚

2. Our team has been working tirelessly to obtain the necessary _____ to ensure our medication is safe and effective for patients.

3. Before a new drug can be marketed, it must undergo rigorous testing and _____ regulatory approval by the appropriate government agencies.

4. This _____ medication has undergone rigorous testing and is now available through our licensed distributors.

5. Pharmacists must be able to _____ between similar sounding drug names to ensure that patients receive the correct medication.

6. Our company has carefully selected a name for our new drug that is _____ to the needs and concerns of our target patient population.

7. Failure to _____ the necessary procedures for drug registration can result in legal consequences for pharmaceutical companies.

8. The drug advertisement was found to be _____ due to its exaggerated claims about the product's effectiveness.

9. The FDA has been _____ in its approval of new drug names, ensuring that they are easy to understand and not confusing for patients.

10. Drug _____ involves a series of clinical trials and testing before it can be approved by the government.

11. The drug registration agency has implemented a comprehensive _____ system to track the progress of each drug application and ensure timely approval.

12. To ensure safety, it is imperative for drug manufacturers to _____ the established standards of drug registration and quality control.

13. The _____ for false advertising can be severe, including fines and potential legal action.

14. The pharmaceutical company applied for a _____ on their new drug's name to protect it from being used by competitors.

15. The pharmaceutical company disclaimed any _____ for the side effects of their new drug in the advertisement.

II. Word Building

Study the Prefixes，Suffixes and Roots in the following grid，and then provide the corresponding word based on the given definition.

Prefixes	Meaning	Example
non-	"not" or "without"（非;无;否定）	nonproprietary
mis-	"wrong"（错;误）	misleading
in-	"not" or "without"（非;无;否定）	ineffective
Suffixes		
-able	"capable of"（能够的;有能力的）	interchangeable
-ive	"having the quality of" or "tending to"（具有……性质的）	attractive
Roots		
sens	"to feel" or "to perceive"（感觉;敏感）	sensitive
intellect	"the faculty of understanding and reasoning"（智力）	intellectual
surveil	"to observe closely" or "to keep watch over"（细察;监视）	surveillance

1. involving the use of natural products and energy in a way that does not harm the environment _____

2. a person who has been chosen to speak or vote for somebody else or on behalf of a group _____

3. having no interesting or unusual features or qualities _____

4. connected with your physical senses _____

5. without limits；without end _____

6. to estimate an amount, a figure, a measurement, etc. wrongly _____

7. a person who places a high value on intellectual pursuits and the development of the mind _____

8. a term that can be used to describe a person or system that is responsible for monitoring, observing, or keeping watch over someone or something _____

9. not safe or protected _____

10. making a strong or vivid impression _____

III. Structure & Function

In English sentences, the past participle（过去分词）and its phrases can function not only as verb tenses of perfect aspect and passive voice, but also as attributive or complement modifiers of nouns and pronouns. For example：

Drug manufacturers must comply with labeling requirements, including providing clear and accurate information about the product's intended use and any potential side effects.

The patent name is the proprietary name used by the manufacturer to protect their intellectual property rights.

The manufacturer may be held liable for any harm caused by their drug if it is found to be unsafe or ineffective.

The World Health Organization requires an INN only for trade names approved in at least two countries worldwide.

Past participle phrases are often used as adverbials in sentences, indicating the meaning of time, reason, conditions, concessions, etc. For example：

Reason：*Diagnosed with a rare disease, the patient was referred to a specialist for further evaluation.*

Condition：*Given more time, the surgeons might have been able to complete the operation successfully.*

Concession：*Told that the project was running behind schedule, they still managed to complete it on time.*

Overall, the use of past participle phrases in medical literature can enhance clarity, objectivity, emphasis, and specificity, ultimately leading to a more effective communication of medical information to readers.

Translate the following sentences, using in each a past participle phrase as an adverbial.

1. 该研究历时两年,揭示了新药人体试验存在的重大伦理问题。

_____

_____

2. 尽管得到 FDA 的批准,但由于潜在的风险,该药物仍然面临法律挑战。

3. 从法律角度来看,必须仔细审查制药公司对其产品不良反应的赔偿责任。

4. 迫于公众对更大透明度的要求,监管机构最近实施了更严格的批准新药的指导方针。

5. 由于担心潜在的副作用,监管机构决定暂停该药物的流通,直到进行进一步的调查。

IV. Audio-visual Exercise

A. Sentence Dictation

Please listen to each sentence twice. First listening is for you to understand the general meaning of the sentence. Try to repeat the sentence after you listen to it for a second time, and then write down the whole sentence during the pauses. You'll listen to all the sentences for a third time for checking your dictation.

1. A drug

2. The name

3. The brand-name

4. The patent name

5. The generic name

B. Visual Comprehension

Watch a video clip three times and decide whether each of the following statements is true（T）or false（F）.

_____ 1. Drug makers in the U. S. nearly doubled their spending on their drug advertisements in 2002.

_____ 2. There is no question that ads for some drugs have been misleading.

_____ 3. Vytorin DTC ads were misleading because they overstated the drug's benefits.

_____ 4. Ads use subtle techniques to ensure that consumers remember the drug's risks rather than benefits.

_____ 5. When detailing risks, ads tend to use faster and more complicated language as well as visual distractions.

_____ 6. There has been for a long time a balance between the presentation of the risks and the benefits in those ads.

_____ 7. The drug industry insists that the best prescription is tighter controls on drug ads.

V. Extended Reading

Read the following dialogue between Dr. Pharmed, a pharmacist and a Food and Drug Administration（FDA）official about drug registration procedures, and complete each statement with a proper phrase or sentence given in the box.

Dr. Pharmed: Good morning, I am Dr. Pharmed, a pharmacist and I would like to inquire about the drug registration procedures.

FDA Official: Good morning, what information are you looking for specifically?

Dr. Pharmed: I would like to know the requirements for registering a new drug with the FDA.

FDA Official: Sure, there are several requirements that must be met before a drug can be registered with the FDA. Firstly, the drug must undergo clinical trials to prove its safety and efficacy. Secondly, the manufacturer must submit an Investigational New Drug（IND）application to the FDA, which includes detailed information about the drug's development, manufacturing, and testing plans. Once the IND is approved, the manufacturer can begin clinical trials. After successful completion of the trials, the manufacturer must submit a New Drug Application (NDA) to the FDA, which includes all data from the clinical trials and additional information about the drug's labeling and proposed use. The NDA is then reviewed by the FDA's Center for Drug Evaluation and Research (CDER), and if approved, the drug can be registered with the FDA.

Dr. Pharmed: Thank you for explaining that. What is the timeline for these procedures?

FDA Official: The timeline varies depending on several factors such as the complexity of the drug and the number of clinical trials required. Generally, it can take several years from the initial submission of an IND to the final registration of a drug with the FDA.

Dr. Pharmed: Is there any assistance available for manufacturers who are unfamiliar with the registration process?

FDA Official: Yes, there are several resources available to help manufacturers navigate the drug registration process. The FDA provides guidance documents and forms on their website, and manufacturers can also seek assistance from consulting firms or professional organizations that specialize in drug development and regulatory affairs.

Dr. Pharmed: That's helpful to know. Thank you for your time and expertise.

FDA Official: You're welcome. If you have any further questions, please don't hesitate to contact us.

1. The drug must _____ to prove its safety and efficacy.
2. An IND application to the FDA should _____ .
3. The manufacture must _____ to the FDA.
4. The timeline for registering a new drug varies _____ .
5. The FDA _____ on their websites.

A. undergo clinical trials

B. submit a New Drug Application (NDA)

C. provides guidance documents and forms

D. seek assistance from consulting firms or professional organizations

E. include detailed information about the drug's development, manufacturing, and testing plans

F. include all data from the clinical trials and additional information about the drug's labeling and proposed use

G. depending on several factors such as the complexity of the drug and the number of clinical trials required

VI. Topics for Discussion and Essay-writing

1. Please explain briefly the differences between a drug's generic name, patent name, and brand-name.

2. What are the principles to which naming a drug should conform?

3. What legal issues may drug advertisements get involved in?

5.4   Drug Pricing

When determining the price of a drug, several factors should be taken into account, including:

R&D costs: The development and testing of a new drug can be expensive, and these costs must be reflected in the price.

Marketing expenses: Drug companies also **incur** significant marketing expenses to **promote** their products, including advertising and **distribution**.

Competition: The price of a drug is often influenced by the prices of similar drugs on the market. If there are many competing drugs available, the price of the drug may need to be lower to remain **competitive**.

Generic competition: If a generic **version** of the drug becomes available, it may reduce the demand for the brand-name drug, leading to lower prices.

Consumer demand: The price of a drug may be affected by consumer demand, as higher-priced drugs may **appeal to** consumers who are willing to pay more for **premium** products.

Government regulations: The government may set

1. Why is it a complex issue to determine the price of a drug?

2. What major factors are to be taken into account when determining the price of a drug?

3. Where does competition arise?

4. How does consumer demand affect the price of a drug?

---

incur /ɪnˈkɜːr/ vt.   招致;引起;遭受
promote /prəˈməʊt/ v.   促进;促销;晋升
distribution /ˌdɪstrɪˈbjuːʃn/ n.   分配;分布;分销
competition /ˌkɒmpəˈtɪʃn/ n.   竞争;比赛;竞争者;竞争产品
competitive /kəmˈpetətɪv/ adj.   竞争的;有竞争力的
version /ˈvɜːrʒn/ n.   版本;变体
appeal to   吸引;呼吁;上诉
premium /ˈpriːmɪəm/ adj.   优质的;高昂的

pricing guidelines for drugs based on various factors, such as **affordability** or **accessibility**.

Overall, pricing a drug involves balancing the costs of development and production with consumer demand and market competition to ensure that the product is both profitable and **accessible** to those who need it.

5.5 Quality of Drugs

The quality of drugs refers to the degree of effectiveness, safety, and purity of a drug. It is an important issue because drugs are used to treat a wide range of illnesses and conditions, and their quality can have a significant impact on the health outcomes of patients.

Effectiveness refers to how well the drug works in treating the intended condition or illness. A high-quality drug should be effective for the target population and have a good safety profile.

Safety refers to the risk of adverse reactions or side effects associated with taking the drug. A high-quality drug should be safe for use and have minimal risks of serious side effects.

Purity refers to the **accuracy** and **consistency** of

1. *What is meant by the quality of drugs?*

2. *Why is the quality of drugs an important issue?*

3. *What is the effectiveness of a drug?*

4. *What does drug safety refer to?*

5. *What does drug purity mean?*

---

affordability /əˌfɔːdəˈbɪlətɪ/ *n.*	支付能力；承受能力；可购性	
accessibility /əkˌsesəˈbɪlətɪ/ *n.*	易接近；可到达；可达性	
accessible /əkˈsesəbl/ *adj.*	可使用的；可进入的；可理解的	
purity /ˈpjʊrətɪ/ *n.*	纯度；纯洁；纯净	
accuracy /ˈækjərəsɪ/ *n.*	精确(性)，准确(性)；准确无误	
consistency /kənˈsɪstənsɪ/ *n.*	连贯性；一致性	

the drug's composition. A high-quality drug should be free from **contaminants** and other **impurities** that could affect its effectiveness or safety.

Overall, ensuring the quality of drugs is critical to protecting patient health and safety. Poor-quality drugs can lead to **suboptimal** treatment outcomes, increase healthcare costs, and even cause harm to patients. Therefore, it is essential to **rigorously** test and regulate the quality of drugs throughout their development, production, and distribution process.

6. Why is it critical to ensure the quality of drugs?

5.6 Intellectual Property Rights of Drugs

Intellectual property rights (IPR) are essential to protect the innovations, discoveries, and creative works of scientists, researchers, and inventors. In the pharmaceutical industry, IPR can refer to various types of legal protection granted to drug products, including patents, trademarks, trade secrets, and **copyrights**. These protections help drugmakers control the distribution and sale of their products while **fostering** innovation and research. However, issues related to IPR in the pharmaceutical industry can also pose significant challenges.

1. What is IPR in the context of pharmaceutical industry?

---

contaminant /kənˈtæmɪnənt/ *n*.　　　　污染物;致污物
impurity /ɪmˈpjʊrətɪ/ *n*.　　　　掺杂;不纯;混杂物;污点
suboptimal /ˈsʌbˈɒptɪməl/ *adj*.　　　未达最佳标准的;不最适宜的;不最满意的
rigorously /ˈrɪgərəslɪ/ *adv*.　　　　严密地;严厉地;残酷地
copyright /ˈkɒpɪraɪt/ *n*.　　　　版权;著作权
foster /ˈfɒstər/ *v*.　　　　促进;鼓励;培养

Patentability: Drugs must undergo a lengthy and expensive process to obtain patents. This can deter drug development by requiring **substantial** investments before any potential benefits are recouped. Additionally, the high cost of obtaining patents can limit access to life-saving treatments for people in low-income countries or those without sufficient resources.

2. What challenges are to be overcome to obtain a drug patent?

Monopolies: Excessive intellectual property protection can lead to monopolies that **stifle** competition and innovation. When a single company holds a majority of patents or trademarks in a particular field, it can prevent smaller companies from entering the market or developing new treatments. This can **hinder** progress in the search for new drugs and treatments for diseases.

3. What can excessive intellectual property protection lead to?

4. What are downsides of monopolies?

Piracy and **counterfeiting**: The **illegal** production and distribution of counterfeit drugs present significant health risks for patients. Piracy and counterfeiting can result in the use of **expired** or **substandard** drugs, which can be harmful or ineffective. This problem is further compounded by the global nature of the pharmaceutical supply chain, making it difficult to **track**

5. Why do counterfeit drugs present significant health risks for patients?

---

patentability /peɪtəntəˈbɪlɪtɪ/ *n*.	专利性
substantial /səbˈstænʃl/ *adj*.	大量的；重大的；结实的
monopoly /məˈnɒpəlɪ/ *n*.	垄断；专卖；垄断者；专利品
stifle /ˈstaɪfl/ *v*.	遏制；扼杀；镇压
hinder /ˈhɪndər/ *v*.	阻碍；妨碍；成为阻碍
piracy /ˈpaɪrəsɪ/ *n*.	盗版行为；非法复制；海上抢劫
counterfeiting /ˈkaʊntəfɪtɪŋ/ *n*.	伪造
illegal /ɪˈliːgl/ *adj*.	不合法的
expired /ɪksˈpaɪəd/ *adj*.	过期的；失效的
substandard /sʌbˈstændərd/ *adj*.	不够标准的；在标准以下的；低等级标准

down and **prosecute perpetrators**.

Trade secrets and **confidential** information: Drugmakers often keep sensitive information about their research and clinical trials confidential to protect their competitive **edge**. However, this **confidentiality** can sometimes extend to unintended consequences, such as the misuse of trade secrets by **competitors** or **malicious** actors seeking to **exploit** confidential information for their own benefit.

Ethical considerations: The commercialization of certain drug compounds or technologies raises ethical questions about the appropriate use of IPR. For example, some argue that certain compounds should be available only through traditional methods of discovery, such as academic research or small-scale manufacturing, rather than being developed **solely** for commercial purposes.

To address these issues, **policymakers** and **stakeholders** in the pharmaceutical industry must strike a balance between protecting intellectual property rights and promoting innovation, access, and fair competition.

6. Why do drugmakers have to keep trade secrets and confidential information?

7. What other ethical issues are involved in the appropriate use of IPR?

---

track down	追查出;追寻;查获
prosecute /ˈprɒsɪkjuːt/ v.	控告;起诉;继续从事;担任控方律师
perpetrator /ˈpɜːpətreɪtə(r)/ n.	做坏事者;犯罪者;行凶者
confidential /ˌkɒnfɪˈdenʃl/ adj.	机密的;保密的;悄悄的
edge /edʒ/ n.	边线;优势;影响力
confidentiality /ˌkɒnfɪˌdenʃɪˈæləti/ n.	机密性
competitor /kəmˈpetɪtər/ n.	竞争者;选手
malicious /məˈlɪʃəs/ adj.	恶意的;有敌意的;蓄意的
exploit /ɪkˈsplɔɪt, ˈeksplɔɪt/ v.	利用;剥削;开采
solely /ˈsəʊlli/ adv.	唯一地;仅仅
policymaker /ˈpɒləsɪˌmeɪkə/ n.	政策制订者;决策人
stakeholder /ˈsteɪkhəʊldə(r)/ n.	股东;利益相关者

This may involve **implementing reforms** to patent laws，encouraging **collaboration** among researchers，**strengthening** international cooperation to **combat** piracy and counterfeiting，and promoting **transparency** around the development and commercialization of new drugs．

8. How can the IPR protection be balanced with the promotion of innovation?

Language Practice

I. Vocabulary Work

Complete each of the following sentences with a suitable word or expression given below．

promote	accessible	substantial	track down
distribution	consistency	monopoly	confidential
appeal to	contaminant	stifle	malicious
premium	impurity	hinder	exploit
affordability	rigorously	strengthen	implement

1. Patients with chronic illnesses often _____ their healthcare providers to recommend more cost-effective alternatives to expensive drugs.

2. Drug manufacturers must ensure that they do not _____ their intellectual property rights by blocking access to essential medications through overpricing or restrictive licensing practices.

3. The expiration of a drug's patent can lead to the development of _____ competition in the market，as other manufacturers enter the space with potentially cheaper versions of the medication.

---

implement /ˈɪmplɪment，ˈɪmplɪmənt/ *v*.　　　实施；执行；使生效
reform /rɪˈfɔːrm/ *n*.　　　改革；改善
collaboration /kəˌlæbəˈreɪʃn/ *n*.　　　协作；合作
strengthen /ˈstreŋθn/ *v*.　　　巩固；加强；增强
combat /ˈkɒmbæt/ *v*.　　　战斗；防止；减轻
transparency /trænsˈpærənsɪ/ *n*.　　　透明；透明度；透明性

4. To ensure the safety and efficacy of drugs, pharmaceutical companies must _____ test their products through clinical trials and other quality control measures.

5. Price negotiation and volume discounts can be used to _____ cost-effective drug pricing, especially for high-volume medications used by a large number of patients.

6. Excessive protection of intellectual property rights in the pharmaceutical industry can _____ research and development, as it may prevent others from accessing and improving upon existing drugs.

7. The pharmaceutical company decided to _____ strict measures to protect their intellectual property rights of drugs from unauthorized use.

8. Ensuring that drugs are _____ to patients in rural and underserved areas is a key aspect of ensuring equitable access to healthcare.

9. Some drugs, especially those that offer novel therapies or treatments for rare diseases, may command a _____ price due to their unique value and the high costs of research and development.

10. The FDA is working closely with law enforcement agencies to investigate reports of _____ attacks on the intellectual property rights of drugs, aiming to ensure the safety and efficacy of medications on the market.

11. The patent system in the pharmaceutical industry has created a _____ on certain drugs, allowing a few companies to control the market and set prices at levels that may not be affordable for all patients.

12. Pharmaceutical companies often have to protect _____ information related to their drug formulas and research, as this intellectual property is crucial to their competitive edge in the market.

13. The drug manufacturer is exploring different _____ channels to reach a wider customer base and potentially reduce drug prices through economies of scale.

14. The abuse of intellectual property rights by some pharmaceutical companies can _____ the availability and affordability of drugs in developing countries, where access to healthcare is already limited.

15. Strict quality control measures are essential to ensure that drugs are free from _____ such as bacteria, viruses, and other microbial impurities.

II. Word Building

Study the Prefixes，*Suffixes and Roots in the following grid*，*and then provide the corresponding word based on the given definition*.

Prefixes	Meaning	Example
sub-	"below or beneath"（低于;在……之下）	substandard
im-	"not" or "lacking"（否定;不;缺乏）	impurity
Suffixes		
-abiliy	"the quality or state of being capable of"（能力）	affordability
-ible	"capable of" or "able to"（能够的）	accessible
-cy	"the quality or state of"（性质;状态）	accuracy
Roots		
mal	"bad" or "evil"（坏;恶）	malicious
access	"to approach" or "to gain access to"（接近;得到）	accessibility
contam	"to soil" or "to make dirty"（弄脏）	contaminant

1. the ability to afford something without causing financial strain _____
2. something that is safe to eat and not poisonous _____
3. accountable, or reliable for their actions or decisions _____
4. something that contaminates _____
5. something that is easily reached, entered, understood, or obtained _____
6. the precision and reliability of facts, data, or details provided in a report, document, or communication _____
7. a secondary title or explanatory text placed below a main title _____
8. a lack of balance or equilibrium, indicating that something is not distributed or proportioned _____
9. a failure to work properly
10. intending to do harm without just cause _____

III. Structure & Function

In English, there are many ways to express the concept of "reason," depending on the specific context and the nuances of meaning that the author wants to convey. For example:

The quality of drugs is an important issue <u>because</u> drugs are used to treat a wide range of illnesses and conditions, and their quality can have a significant impact on the health outcomes of patients.

The price of a drug may be affected by consumer demand, <u>as</u> higher-priced drugs may appeal to consumers who are willing to pay more for premium products.

<u>Since</u> the side effects were minimal, we concluded that the drug was safe for human consumption.

<u>As a result of</u> the study, we discovered that the drug was effective in treating the targeted condition.

<u>Owing to</u> the drug's unique mechanism of action, it has the potential to revolutionize the treatment of the disease.

<u>On account of</u> the positive results from the preclinical studies, we initiated the process of filing for regulatory approval.

The delay in the approval process for our new drug is <u>due to</u> the rigorous testing required by the FDA.

Translate the following sentences, using in each an expression given in parentheses.

1. 试验失败的原因是治疗组中副作用发生率较高,这是由于药物的毒性所导致的。(as a result of)

_____

_____

2. 既然当前的治疗方案未能达到预期效果,公司决定投资研究替代治疗方案。(since)

_____

_____

3. 由于初步研究结果很有前景,我们决定进一步投资于该潜在药物的研发。(owing to)

_____

_____

4. 由于新药在临床试验中表现出良好的效果,我们决定继续推进下一阶段的研发工作。(on account of)

_____

_____

5. 由于药物在患者疗效方面表现出显著改善,我们决定继续进行第三阶段的临床试验。(as)

_____

_____

IV. Audio-visual Exercise

A. Sentence Dictation

Please listen to each sentence twice. First listening is for you to understand the general meaning of the sentence. Try to repeat the sentence after you listen to it for a second time，and then write down the whole sentence during the pauses. You'll listen to all the sentences for a third time for checking your dictation.

1. Advertising a drug _____

_____

2. A high-quality drug _____

_____

3. Drug effectiveness _____

_____

4. Drug safety _____

_____

5. The legal requirements _____

_____

B. Visual Comprehension

Watch a video three times and decide whether each of the following statements is true（T）or false（F）.

_____ 1. There was doubt whether generic drugs are truly identical to brand-name drugs in terms of effectiveness and safety.

_____ 2. Sassee Ann Arnold had a bad reaction to a generic drug when she received a generic version.

_____ 3. According to Dr. Janet Woodcock from the FDA, the majority of Americans are not satisfied with generic drugs.

_____ 4. Generic drugs are required to contain the exact same amount of active ingredient as the original.

_____ 5. The filler ingredients in generic drugs are no different from those in the brand-name drugs.

_____ 6. Most prescription medications are generics and the majority of them have no problems.

_____ 7. The video clip is mainly about why generic drugs are cheaper than brand-name drugs.

V. Extended Reading

Read the following dialogue between Dr. Pharmed and students about drug quality issues, and complete the dialogue with a suitable phrase or sentence from the grid.

Dr. Pharmed: Good morning, everybody. Today, we'll be discussing drug quality issues. Can anyone tell me what are some of the most common issues related to drug quality?

Student 1: I think that one of the biggest issues is contamination. Sometimes drugs can __1__, which can affect their safety and effectiveness.

Dr. Pharmed: That's a good point. Contamination is a major concern for both patients and healthcare providers. In addition to affecting drug safety, it can also lead to adverse reactions in some cases. It's important for manufacturers to __2__.

Student 2: What about drug counterfeiting? How does that impact drug quality?

Dr. Pharmed: Yes, drug counterfeiting is another significant issue related to drug quality. When a patient receives a counterfeit medication, they may not receive the same level of efficacy or safety as they would from a genuine product. Additionally, counterfeit drugs can __3__, which can be dangerous for patients. Manufacturers and regulatory agencies work together to combat counterfeiting by implementing strict packaging and labeling requirements, as well as tracking and monitoring the supply chain for counterfeit products.

Student 3: Are there any other issues related to drug quality?

Dr. Pharmed: Yes, there are many other issues related to drug quality. For example, some drugs can __4__. Others may have unintended side effects or interactions with other medications. It's important for healthcare providers to monitor patients' responses to treatments and report any concerns related to drug quality to their prescribing physician. This helps ensure that patients __5__ and that potential risks are identified and addressed promptly.

Student 4: What role do patients play in ensuring drug quality?

Dr. Pharmed: Patient involvement is critical in ensuring drug quality. Patients can help by following their prescribed regimen carefully and reporting any adverse reactions or concerns related to their treatment to their healthcare provider. They can also __6__ by asking questions and staying informed about the latest developments in their condition. By working together, patients and healthcare providers can help ensure that patients receive high-quality medications that provide the best possible outcomes.

Student 5: Thank you for your time today. It's important for us as healthcare professionals to stay up-to-date on these issues so that we can __7__.

Dr. Pharmed: You're absolutely right! Staying informed about drug quality issues is essential for ensuring that patients receive the best possible care.

_____	1	A. receive the best possible care
_____	2	B. advocate for safe and effective medications
_____	3	C. provide our patients with safe and effective treatments
_____	4	D. have a significant impact on the health outcomes of patients

_____ 5	E. contain harmful ingredients or be adulterated with other substances
_____ 6	F. lose their potency over time due to changes in temperature or storage conditions
_____ 7	G. implement rigorous quality control measures to minimize the risk of contamination
	H. become contaminated with other substances during production or packaging

VI. Topics for Discussion and Essay-writing

1. What factors do pharmaceutical companies take into account when pricing the new drugs they develop?

2. Should the government propose guidelines for drug pricing? Why?

3. How to balance the relationship between protecting intellectual property rights and promoting innovation and fair competition?

5.7 Animal Testing

Animal testing for drugs is a **controversial** issue with ethical concerns. Some people argue that animal testing is necessary to ensure the safety and effectiveness of new drugs, while others believe that it is **inhumane** and unnecessary. There are several ethical concerns associated with animal testing for drugs, including:

Animal **welfare**: Animals used for drug testing may experience pain, suffering, and death, which raises concerns about their welfare.

1. Why is animal testing for drugs a controversial issue?

Ethical **implications**: Animal testing for drugs raises ethical questions about the value of animal life and the potential harm caused to animals.

2. What ethical questions are raised by animal testing for drugs?

Alternatives: There are alternative methods of drug testing that do not involve animal testing, such as computer **modeling**, **in vitro** testing, and human clinical trials.

3. What are the alternative to animal testing for drugs?

Regulatory requirements: In some countries, there are strict regulatory requirements for animal testing, such as the use of **humanely** raised animals and the **provision** of **adequate** care during testing.

---

controversial /ˌkɒntrəˈvɜːʃl/ adj.	有争议的;引发争论的
inhumane /ˌɪnhjuːˈmeɪn/ adj.	残忍的;不人道的
welfare /ˈwelfeə(r)/ n.	幸福;安全与健康;福利
implication /ˌɪmplɪˈkeɪʃn/ n.	可能的影响;含意;牵连
modeling /ˈmɒdlɪŋ/ n.	建模;造型(术)
in vitro /ɪnˈviːtrəʊ/	在生物体外进行的;用试管进行的
humanely /hjuːˈmeɪnlɪ/ adv.	人道地;慈悲地
provision /prəˈvɪʒn/ n.	提供;供给
adequate /ˈædɪkwət/ adj.	足够的;合格的;合乎需要的

Overall, the use of animals for drug testing is a complex issue with both ethical and practical considerations. It is important to carefully weigh the potential benefits and risks of animal testing when making decisions about its use in drug development.

4. Why is it important to weigh carefully the the potential benefits and risks of animal testing for drugs?

5.8   Research Integrity

Drug research **integrity** refers to the ethical and scientific principles that must be followed when conducting drug research to ensure the **legitimacy**, **authenticity**, and **reproducibility** of the research results. These principles include the following:

1. What constitutes the core of drug research integrity?

Scientific **hypothesis** and purpose: The research hypothesis must be well-founded and **purposeful**, and the research must have scientific basis and theoretical support.

2. What is said about the research hypothesis?

Data authenticity and reproducibility: The data must be **authentic**, accurate, and **reliable**, and the results must be **reproducible**. Any data **falsification**, **fabrication**,

3. What do data authenticity and reproducibility mean?

---

integrity /ɪnˈtegrətɪ/ *n*.　　　　　正直,诚实;完整
legitimacy /lɪˈdʒɪtɪməsɪ/ *n*.　　　　合法(性);合理(性);正当(性)
authenticity /ˌɔːθenˈtɪsətɪ/ *n*.　　　真实性;可靠性;确实性
reproducibility /rɪprədjuːsəˈbɪlɪtɪ/ *n*.　再现性;复现性;可重现性
hypothesis /haɪˈpɒθəsɪs/ *n*.　　　　　假设;假说;猜想;猜测
purposeful /ˈpɜːpəsfl/ *adj*.　　　　　有明确目的的;故意的;果断的
authentic /ɔːˈθentɪk/ *adj*.　　　　　真实的;逼真的
reliable /rɪˈlaɪəbl/ *adj*.　　　　　　可靠的;可信赖的;真实可信的
reproducible /ˌrɪprəˈdjʊsəbl/ *adj*.　　可复现的;可再生的
falsification /ˌfɔːlsɪfɪˈkeɪʃn/ *n*.　　　伪造;弄虚作假;篡改
fabrication /ˌfæbrɪˈkeɪʃn/ *n*.　　　　捏造;编造;制造;生产

or inappropriate **interpolation** or interpolation for ill purposes is **unethical** and illegal.

Animal ethics and human rights：Animal ethics and human rights principles must be followed during drug research. The researchers must respect the rights of animals and use them in an appropriate way，while respecting human rights，including respecting patients' privacy，protecting patients' personal information，and obtaining **informed consent** from patients.

4. *What does respecting human rights mean in drug research?*

Conflict of interest **disclosure**：Researchers must disclose any conflicts of interest，including financial relationships with drug companies or other organizations that may have an interest in the research results. This ensures that the research is **objective** and **independent**.

5. *Why is disclosing interest conflicts essential in maintaining drug research integrity?*

Intellectual property protection：Intellectual property protection must be followed during drug research to ensure that the results of the research are protected and can be used for future development and innovation.

6. *Why must intellectual property protection be followed during drug research?*

Ethical review and **supervision**：Drug research projects must undergo ethical review and supervision to ensure that the research meets ethical standards and legal requirements. This review should be independent, blind，and reliable to ensure that the review results are objective and accurate.

7. *Why must drug research projects undergo ethical review and supervision?*

---

interpolation /ɪnˌtɜːpəˈleɪʃn/ n .   插值；内插；补充部分
unethical /ʌnˈeθɪkl/ adj .   不道德的
informed /ɪnˈfɔːmd/ adj .   了解情况的；有见识的；有根据的
consent /kənˈsent/ n .   准许；同意；赞同
conflict /ˈkɒnflɪkt/ n .   冲突；争执；战斗；矛盾
disclosure /dɪsˈkləʊʒə(r)/ n .   公开；披露；揭露
objective /əbˈdʒektɪv/ adj ./n .   客观的；基于事实的；目标；目的
independent /ˌɪndɪˈpendənt/ adj .   不相关的；不受影响的；独立的
supervision /ˌsjuːpəˈvɪʒn/ n .   监督；管理

5.9   Marketing Ethics

Drug marketing ethics refers to the principles that guide the way in which drugs are marketed and sold to the public. These principles are intended to ensure that drug marketing is conducted in a responsible and ethical manner, with the **primary** goal of promoting the safety and effectiveness of drugs while minimizing any potential harms or risks.

1. What are the primary objectives of drug marketing ethics?

There are several key aspects of drug marketing ethics that should be considered.

Firstly, drug companies must ensure that their marketing activities are **truthful** and not misleading. This means that they must provide accurate information about the drugs they are selling, including their potential side effects and benefits, and avoid making false or **exaggerated** claims about their efficacy.

2. What is the first drug marketing ethics to be considered?

Secondly, drug companies must respect the privacy and confidentiality of their patients. This means that they must obtain informed consent from patients before collecting any personal data, and keep this information secure and confidential. They must also respect patients' rights to **access** and control their medical records, and not disclose this information without their consent.

3. What is meant by respecting the privacy and confidentiality of the patients?

Thirdly, drug companies must take into account

---

primary /ˈpraɪmərɪ/ *adj*.　　首要的;最早的;初级的
truthful /ˈtruːθfl/ *adj*.　　真实的;如实的;诚实的
exaggerated /ɪɡˈzædʒəreɪtɪd/ *adj*.　　夸大的;言过其实的
access /ˈækses/ *v*.　　获取;获得;访问

the social and cultural context in which their drugs are being marketed. This means that they must be sensitive to issues such as race, **gender**, age, and **sexual orientation**, and avoid any marketing activities that may be **offensive** or **discriminatory** to certain groups of people.

Finally, drug companies must ensure that their marketing activities do not exploit **vulnerable** populations, such as young people or individuals who are already taking multiple medications. This means that they must be careful not to promote their drugs in ways that could be harmful or **addictive** to these individuals, and must work to raise awareness about the potential risks associated with drug use.

Overall, drug marketing ethics is an important issue that affects the health and well-being of people around the world. By following these principles, drug companies can help to promote the safety and effectiveness of their products while minimizing any potential harms or risks.

4. What social and cultural issues must drug companies be sensitive to?

5. How should drug companies avoid exploiting vulnerable populations?

6. What can drug companies benefit from following these marketing principles?

Language Practice

I. Vocabulary Work

Complete each of the following sentences with a suitable word or expression given

gender /ˈdʒendə(r)/ *n.*	性别
sexual /ˈsekʃuəl/ *adj.*	性的;与性别有关的;有关性行为的
orientation /ˌɔːriənˈteɪʃn/ *n.*	方向;取向;目标;观点态度
offensive /əˈfensɪv/ *adj.*	无礼冒犯的;令人不快的;攻击的
discriminatory /dɪˈskrɪmɪnətərɪ/ *adj.*	歧视性的;区别对待的;不公平的
vulnerable /ˈvʌlnərəbl/ *adj.*	易受伤害的;脆弱的
addictive /əˈdɪktɪv/ *adj.*	使人成瘾的;使人入迷的

below.

controversial	provision	authentic	consent
vulnerable	adequate	reliable	conflicts
implications	integrity	fabrication	disclosure
supervision	legitimacy	unethical	access
discriminatory	hypothesis	informed	offensive

1. The _____ of pharmaceutical research and development is underpinned by adherence to rigorous scientific methodologies, ethical standards, and regulatory compliance, ensuring that the drugs brought to market are safe and efficacious.

2. The marketing and distribution strategies employed by pharmaceutical companies should also not be _____ , ensuring that new medications reach underserved communities and do not perpetuate existing health disparities based on socioeconomic status, race, or gender.

3. Maintaining the highest levels of scientific _____ throughout the drug development process ensures that clinical trials adhere to rigorous standards, leading to trustworthy and reliable results which regulatory agencies can use to approve or deny market access.

4. _____ consent is a fundamental principle in pharmaceutical research and development, where participants must be fully informed about the nature of the study, potential risks and benefits, before deciding to participate.

5. The process of drug approval often necessitates full _____ of clinical trial data, including adverse events and limitations of the study, to regulatory agencies for thorough evaluation and to ensure public safety.

6. Data _____ in pharmaceutical research and development is a serious ethical violation that undermines the integrity of scientific findings, potentially leading to unsafe drugs being approved or effective treatments being withheld from patients.

7. The use of _____ samples from patients is essential for drug discovery and development.

8. In pharmaceutical research and development, _____ populations such as children, pregnant women, and the elderly are often excluded from clinical trials due to safety concerns; however, their unique needs must be considered when developing appropriate dosages and formulations.

9. In drug marketing, it's essential to avoid language or terminology that could be considered _____ by patients or communities, especially when discussing sensitive health conditions or cultural beliefs related to medicine.

10. In pharmaceutical research and development, rigorous _____ is critical to ensure that all experiments and clinical trials are conducted in accordance with established ethical guidelines, good laboratory practices (GLP), and good clinical practices (GCP).

11. Falsifying data, manipulating test results, or fabricating research findings are egregious examples of _____ conduct in pharmaceutical R&D that not only tarnish the reputation of the individuals involved but also undermine the trust in scientific research and harm public health.

12. Open-_____ policies for research data and publications are becoming increasingly important in pharmaceutical R&D, allowing scientists worldwide to build upon existing knowledge, accelerate discovery, and ultimately improve patient access to cutting-edge therapies.

13. _____ over intellectual property rights are common in pharmaceutical R&D, especially when multiple parties claim ownership or rights to a particular drug compound, manufacturing process, or innovative technology.

14. The discovery of unforeseen side effects in early stages of pharmaceutical research and development can have significant _____ for the drug's safety profile, potentially leading to changes in its chemical structure or even termination of the project.

15. In drug research, a _____ is the cornerstone of every drug discovery project; it represents the scientist's initial theory about how a compound might interact with a biological system to produce a therapeutic effect.

II. Word Building

Study the Prefixes，Suffixes and Roots in the following grid，and then provide the corresponding word based on the given definition.

Prefixes	**Meaning**	**Example**
dis-	"not" or "opposite of"（否定或相反）	disclosure
un-	"not" or "opposite of"（否定或相反）	unethical
hypo-	"under，beneath or less than"（在……下面；低于）	hypothesis
Suffixes		
-ful	"full of"（充满）	truthful
-sion	"the action or process of ……"（动作或过程）	provision
-ure	"a state or condition of"（状态或情况）	disclosure
Roots		
legit	"lawful" or ""authorized by law"（合法的；法律允许的）	legitimacy
sent	"to feel or think"（感觉或思考）	consent

1. giving the true facts about something _____

2. morally wrong and unacceptable according to rules or beliefs about morality

   _____

3. recognized or accepted as legal or valid; lawful _____

4. a feeling or an opinion, especially one based on emotions _____

5. an idea that is based on a few known facts but that has not yet been proved to be true or correct _____

6. to make something lawful or acceptable; to validate _____

7. the act of making new or secret information known _____

8. the state of being exposed to something _____

9. the act of supplying somebody with something that they need or want _____

10. agreement or permission given voluntarily by someone who has the power or authority to grant it _____

III. Structure & Function

An elliptical sentence（省略句）is a sentence in which some words are omitted for brevity or grammatical reasons. Elliptical sentences introduced by conjunctions like when, while, if, or unless can be used to create a more complex sentence structure that conveys multiple ideas or conditions. This type of sentence is often used in medical English to provide additional information or clarification about the conditions under which a treatment or intervention is safe or effective. For example:

It is important to carefully weigh the potential benefits and risks of animal testing <u>when making decisions about its use in drug development</u>.

The researchers must respect the rights of animals and use them in an appropriate way, <u>while respecting human rights, including respecting patients' privacy, protecting patients' personal information, and obtaining informed consent from patients</u>.

<u>When confronted with evidence of their wrongdoing</u>, the researcher admitted to falsifying their results.

<u>If conducted ethically</u>, clinical trials can lead to groundbreaking treatments.

<u>Unless guided by ethical principles</u>, drug research can lead to unethical practices.

<u>As seen in the recent scandal</u>, the lack of research integrity can have serious consequences for the entire field of medicine.

One stylistic effect achieved by using elliptical sentences introduced by conjunctions is to create a more formal and precise tone. Another effect is to create a more varied sentence structure, which can make the writing more interesting and engaging for readers. Using conjunctions to introduce elliptical sentences can also help to convey complex ideas or relationships between different factors, such as the relationship between drug development and the potential harms or risks. Overall, using elliptical sentences introduced by conjunctions can help to improve the clarity, precision, and sophistication of medical writing.

Translate the following sentences into English, using in each an elliptical sentence structure introduced by a conjunction.

1. 若得到严格遵守,监管指南可确保药物研究中的患者安全。

_____

_____

2. 除非有透明的数据支持,否则关于新药疗效的声明可能遭到怀疑。

_____   _____

_____

3. 进行实验时,研究人员必须保持警惕以确保他们的方法合乎伦理并且严密。

_____

_____

4. 当被问及其方法时,研究团队无法就其数据收集过程提供令人满意的答复。

_____

_____

5. 如同媒体报道的那样,那两位科学家的研究结果受到质疑,因为发现他们伪造了实验结果。

_____

_____

IV. Audio-visual Exercise

A. Listening Comprehension

Listen to a passage, which will be spoken only once. After you hear the passage, you must choose the best answer to each question from the four choices marked A, B, C, and D.

1. Research integrity is particularly important in drug R&D because it ensures

   _____.

   A. the reliability of the drawn conclusions

   B. the safety and efficacy of new drugs

   C. the accuracy of the generated data

   D. all the above mentioned

2. Which of the following is mentioned as a form of scientific misconduct?

   A. Falsifying data.　　　　　　　　B. Biased analysis.

   C. Inaccurate reporting.　　　　　　D. Nontransparent purpose.

3. Researchers' competence includes their understanding of the following EXCEPT

   _____.

   A. relevant scientific principles

B. regulations governing drug R & D

C. skills to carry out work effectively

D. research methods and procedures

4. The results of drug R & D studies should be _____ .

　　A. publishable

　　B. reproducible

　　C. transparent

　　D. manageable

5. The passage mainly discusses _____ .

　　A. key research principles

　　B. best practices in research

　　C. research data management

　　D. standards of research integrity

B. Visual Comprehension

Watch a video clip three times and complete each of the following statements based on the video you have just watched .

1. A small study made in 1998 by Dr. Andrew Wakefield, a British surgeon and researcher, set off a global public health scare, impacting the way so many parents make decisions about _____ .

2. But a prominent medical journal says Dr. Wakefield's study about a link between the measles, mumps, rubella vaccine and autism was in fact _____

_____ .

3. The investigative reporter Brian Deer debunked Wakefields' study, saying he found Dr. Wakefield falsified _____ .

4. Dan and Kelly Lacek were angry that they didn't vaccinate their youngest son based on a purported fraud, saying that it's been a fraud and that it's _____

_____ .

5. Doctors all over the country are reacting with outrage to news of Dr. Wakefield's alleged fabrications, saying that his study back in 1998 led to a dramatic drop in vaccinations, which provoked more _____ .

V. Extended Reading

Read the following dialogue between Dr . Pharmed and students about issues of intellectual property rights in drug R&D，and choose the best answer to each question according to the dialogue .

Dr. Pharmed: Good morning, everyone. Today, we'll be discussing issues of intellectual property rights in drug R&D. Can anyone tell me what are some of the key concerns related to this topic?

Student 1: I think that one of the biggest issues is the potential for intellectual property theft or infringement by other companies. Sometimes researchers may unknowingly develop a drug that is similar to one developed by a competitor, which could lead to legal disputes and financial losses for both parties.

Dr. Pharmed: That's a good point. Intellectual property theft and infringement can have serious consequences for drug developers and can undermine the progress of medical research. It's important for researchers to protect their intellectual property by obtaining patents and trademarks on their inventions and ensuring that they do not infringe on the intellectual property rights of others. Additionally, regulatory agencies often monitor patent filings to ensure that they are being used appropriately and to prevent potential abuses.

Student 2: What about issues related to open access publishing? How does that impact drug R&D?

Dr. Pharmed: Yes, open access publishing is another significant concern related to intellectual property rights in drug R&D. Open access publishing allows researchers to share their research findings freely online, which can help accelerate the pace of medical discovery and improve patient outcomes. However, open access publishing can also pose challenges for companies developing new drugs, as it may make it easier for competitors to copy their research or identify potential new treatments. Companies may need to balance the benefits of open access publishing with the need to protect their intellectual property and commercialize their discoveries effectively.

Student 3: Are there any other issues related to intellectual property rights in drug R&D?

Dr. Pharmed: Yes, there are many other issues related to intellectual property rights in drug R & D. For example, some researchers may engage in data sharing without proper licensing agreements, which could lead to conflicts over ownership of data generated during drug development. Others may use non-proprietary software or hardware without obtaining proper licenses or permissions, which could lead to legal disputes over intellectual property rights. It's important for researchers and companies to carefully consider the implications of intellectual property rights when conducting drug R & D activities.

Student 4: What role do patients play in ensuring intellectual property rights in drug R & D?

Dr. Pharmed: Patients can help ensure intellectual property rights in drug R & D by supporting policies that promote open access publishing and transparency in scientific research. By advocating for these policies and encouraging their healthcare providers to participate in open access clinical trials, patients can help ensure that new drugs are developed in an ethical and sustainable manner that benefits patients and society as a whole.

Student 5: Thank you for your time today. It's important for us as healthcare professionals to stay up-to-date on these issues so that we can provide our patients with safe and effective treatments based on accurate and reliable information.

Dr. Pharmed: You're absolutely right! Staying informed about issues related to intellectual property rights in drug R & D is essential for ensuring that patients receive the best possible care and that medical research continues to advance in a responsible and ethical manner.

1. According to Dr. Pharmed, intellectual property theft and infringement can _____ .

   A. lead to financial losses for patients

   B. undermine the progress of medical research

   C. result in legal disputes among drug developers

   D. be considered the most important issues in drug R & D

2. What does Dr. Pharmed think of open access publishing?

   A. It can help accelerate the pace of medical discovery.

   B. It allows researchers to share their research findings online.

   C. It is a significant concern which impacts drug R & D negatively.

   D. It brings both benefits and challenges for companies to develop new drugs.

3. What is another issue related to intellectual property rights in drug R & D?

   A. Some researchers may use non-proprietary software or hardware without obtaining proper permissions.

   B. Some researchers may engage in legal disputes over intellectual property rights.

   C. Some conflicts may arise over ownership of data generated during drug development.

   D. Some companies underestimate the implications of intellectual property rights.

4. Patients can play a significant role in ensuring intellectual property rights in drug R & D by _____ .

   A. supporting transparency in scientific research

   B. encouraging an open access clinical trials

   C. promoting open access publishing

   D. doing all of the above mentioned

5. Why is it important for healthcare professionals to be knowledgeable about intellectual property rights in drug R & D?

   A. To ensure that they prescribe drugs with strong IP protections.

   B. To better understand the complex drug development process.

   C. To provide patients with safe, ethical, and reliable treatments.

   D. To avoid inadvertently infringing on the right of their patents.

VI. Topics for Discussion and Essay-writing

1. Why is animal testing for drugs a controversial topic?

2. What are the issues involved in drug research integrity?

3. What ethical issues should be considered in drug marketing?

Chapter VI

Safety Regulation of Drugs

6.1 Implementation of International Pharmaceutical Standards

International pharmaceutical standards refer to a series of guidelines and standards that are established and implemented by the global community for the research, development, production, quality control, and use of pharmaceuticals. These standards are intended to ensure the safety, efficacy, and quality of pharmaceuticals and are primarily intended for protecting public health. International pharmaceutical standards are typically developed and recommended by international organizations such as the World Health Organization (WHO), the International Conference on **Harmonization** of Technical Requirements for Registration of Pharmaceuticals for Human Use (ICH), the European Medicines Agency (EMA), and the United States Food and Drug Administration (FDA).

The implementation of these standards involves a variety of activities, including:

1. What is the purpose of establishing international pharmaceutical standards?

2. What organizations are responsible for developing international pharmaceutical standards?

---

harmonization /ˌhɑːmənaɪˈzeɪʃn/ *n.*　　　　和谐;协调;相称

Regular monitoring of drug manufacturing processes to ensure **compliance** with regulatory requirements.

Inspections of manufacturing **facilities** to assess their compliance with regulations and quality control measures.

Testing of drugs to ensure they meet established safety and efficacy **criteria**.

Review of clinical trials to ensure that they have been conducted in **accordance** with established guidelines.

Collaboration with international organizations and regulatory bodies to share information and best practices.

Implementation of international pharmaceutical standards typically occurs through national regulations and compliance with regional harmonized standards. At the national level, each country has its own regulations and standards that must be met by **domestic** drug manufacturers, research **institutions**, and drug **suppliers**. These regulations and standards cover all aspects of the pharmaceutical industry, including drug research, development, production, quality control, labeling, advertising, sales, and use. The implementation of international pharmaceutical standards also ensures **compatibility** and transparency of technical regulations and standards among countries and regions.

3. What activities occur in the implementation of international pharmaceutical standards?

4. How are international pharmaceutical standards implemented?

---

compliance /kəmˈplaɪəns/ n.	遵守;服从
inspection /ɪnˈspekʃn/ n.	检查;检验;视察
facility /fəˈsɪlətɪ/ n.	设施;才能;天赋
criteria /kraɪˈtɪrɪə/ n.	标准;准则
review /rɪˈvjuː/ n.	评审;检查;评论
accordance /əˈkɔːrdns/ n.	依照;依据;一致
domestic /dəˈmestɪk/ adj.	国内的;家用的;驯养的
institution /ˌɪnstɪˈtuːʃn/ n.	机构;社会收容机构;习俗
supplier /səˈplaɪər/ n.	供应商;供应国;供应者
compatibility /kəmˌpætəˈbɪlətɪ/ n.	并存;相容;兼容性

6.2 Implementation of China's Pharmaceutical Standards

Pharmaceutical standards are a set of regulations and standards formulated and implemented by the Chinese government for the research, development, production, sales, and use of pharmaceuticals. The goal of these standards is to ensure the safety, efficacy, and quality of pharmaceuticals to protect public health.

China's pharmaceutical standards can be divided into two **categories**: national standards and local standards. National standards refer to the national drug standards **formulated** by the Chinese government, including the national drug standard code, drug standards, **specifications** for drug use, etc. Local standards mainly refer to the **provincial** drug standards formulated by local governments based on national standards, including local standards for the use of traditional Chinese medicine, traditional Chinese medicine internal control standard, etc.

China has a comprehensive system of pharmaceutical standards that is implemented through various organizations, including the State Food and Drug Administration (SFDA), China National Standardization Administration (CNAS), and the Chinese Academy of Agricultural Sciences (CAAS).

1. What is the purpose of pharmaceutical standards in China?

2. What are the two categories of pharmaceutical standards in China?

3. How do local standards relate to national standards?

4. What organizations are involved in implementing China's comprehensive system of pharmaceutical standards?

---

category /ˈkætəgɔːrɪ/ n.　　　　种类;类别
formulate /ˈfɔːrmjʊleɪt/ v.　　　构想出;规划;确切地阐述
specification /ˌspesɪfɪˈkeɪʃn/ n.　　规格;详述;说明书
provincial /prəˈvɪnʃəl/ adj.　　　省的;州的;领地的;地方的

The SFDA is responsible for regulating the production, marketing, and distribution of drugs in China. It sets national drug standards, inspects and monitors factories to ensure compliance with these standards, and issues licenses for drug manufacturing and **importation**. These standards cover a wide range of areas, including safety, efficacy, quality, and packaging. The key components of these standards include:

Safety: The standards cover the safety of drugs during their development, testing, manufacturing, marketing, and use.

Efficacy: The standards cover the effectiveness of drugs in treating diseases or conditions.

Quality: The standards cover the quality of drugs, including their purity, potency, and **stability**.

Packaging: The standards cover the packaging of drugs to ensure that they are safe and easy to handle.

Overall, China's pharmaceutical standards are designed to ensure the safety, efficacy, and quality of drugs. The implementation of these standards is **overseen** by a variety of organizations, with strict inspections and monitoring procedures in place to maintain compliance.

In addition to the above standards, there are also some professional association standards and **enterprise** standards formulated by professional associations and pharmaceutical enterprises to ensure the quality and safety of pharmaceuticals.

5. What are the key components of the national drug standards set by the SFDA?

6. What measures are in place to maintain compliance with China's pharmaceutical standards?

---

importation /ˌɪmpɔːˈteʃən/ *n*.　　　　进口;输入;进口货
stability /stəˈbɪlətɪ/ *n*.　　　　　　稳定(性);稳固;坚定
oversee /ˌəʊvərˈsɪ/ *v*.　　　　　　　监督;监视;俯瞰
enterprise /ˈentərpraɪz/ *n*.　　　　公司;企业单位

6.3 Safety Assessment and Quality Control of Drugs

Safety **assessment** of drugs involves a series of steps to evaluate the potential risks associated with a drug and **determine** whether it is safe for use. Some common safety assessment methods include:

1. What is the purpose of drug safety assessment?

Preclinical studies: These are studies conducted in animals or cells before the drug is tested in humans. The goal of these studies is to identify potential toxic or adverse effects of the drug and to assess its safety and efficacy. For example, researchers might conduct preclinical studies on mice to evaluate the safety and efficacy of an Alzheimer's drug before conducting clinical trials in humans.

2. What is the goal of preclinical studies?

Clinical trials: These are studies conducted in humans to evaluate the safety and efficacy of a drug. Clinical trials are divided into several phases, with each phase designed to test different aspects of the drug's safety and efficacy. For example, phase I trials may involve testing the drug on a small group of healthy volunteers to evaluate its safety and dosage requirements, while phase III trials may involve testing the drug on larger groups of people to evaluate its effectiveness and side effects.

3. What is the purpose of each phase in clinical trials?

Post-marketing surveillance: This is a continuous monitoring of drugs after they have been approved for

---

assessment /əˈsesmənt/ *n.*   看法;评估;鉴定

determine /dɪˈtɜːrmɪn/ *v.*   查明;测定;准确算出;决定

use by regulatory agencies. The goal of post-marketing surveillance is to detect any safety issues or adverse reactions that may arise from the use of the drug. This can include monitoring databases for reports of adverse events, conducting ongoing clinical trials to gather additional data, and reviewing patient records to identify any patterns or trends in drug use that may be associated with adverse events.

4. How does post-marketing surveillance help in detecting safety issues or adverse reactions from drugs?

Overall, safety assessment of drugs is a complex and **multidisciplinary** process that involves collaboration between scientists, clinicians, regulators, and other stakeholders. The goal is to ensure that drugs are safe for use and that their benefits **outweigh** their risks.

5. Who are involved in the safety assessment of drugs?

Quality control of drugs involves a series of processes and procedures to ensure that the drugs are safe, effective, and meet established quality standards. Some examples of quality control measures for drugs include:

6. What does quality control of drugs aim to ensure?

Regular monitoring of drug manufacturing processes to ensure compliance with regulatory requirements.

Inspections of manufacturing facilities to assess their compliance with regulations and quality control measures.

Testing of drugs to ensure they meet established safety and efficacy criteria.

Review of clinical trials to ensure that they have been conducted in accordance with established guidelines.

Collaboration with international organizations and regulatory bodies to share information and best practices.

---

multidisciplinary /ˌmʌltɪdɪsəˈplɪnərɪ/ *adj.*   包括各种学科的;多学科的;多部门的
outweigh /ˌaʊtˈweɪ/ *v.*   比……重要;胜过;强过;比……有价值

For example, quality control measures for an Alzheimer's drug might include regular testing of the drug to ensure that it is still effective and safe for use, as well as monitoring for any side effects or adverse reactions. The drug might also be tested on animals or in clinical trials before being approved for use in humans.

Additionally, the manufacturing process for the drug would need to be closely monitored to ensure that it meets strict quality control standards.

In controlled settings, such as hospitals or clinics, quality control is typically performed by healthcare providers or pharmacists who review patients' medication records and monitor the effectiveness of medications. They may also perform routine testing on medications to ensure that they are still effective and safe for use.

7. What type of quality control measures might be implemented for an Alzheimer's drug?

8. What actions do healthcare providers or pharmacists take to monitor the effectiveness of medications?

Language Practice

I. Vocabulary Work

Complete each of the following sentences with a suitable word or expression given below.

compliance	accordance	formulate	oversee
inspection	domestic	specification	enterprise
facility	institution	importation	assessment
criteria	compatibility	component	determine
review	category	stability	outweigh

1. Ensuring _____ with traditional Chinese medicine formulations is a key consideration in pharmaceutical development within the country, as it allows for the integration of novel therapies with existing holistic health practices.

2. International pharmaceutical standards require that all medications adhere to

_____ guidelines which detail the quality, purity, and potency of active ingredients as well as the acceptable limits for impurities.

3. The new manufacturing _____ has been equipped with advanced technology to ensure the production of high-quality medicinal products.

4. The benefits of adopting international pharmaceutical standards in drug safety and assessment _____ the potential costs, as it leads to a more robust and reliable healthcare system.

5. Maintaining the _____ of drugs and assessing their shelf life under different storage conditions is crucial for safety evaluation and quality assurance in pharmaceutical manufacturing.

6. Pharmaceutical companies operating in China are required to adhere to stringent quality control standards in _____ with the National Medical Products Administration guidelines, ensuring that all drug development processes meet rigorous safety and efficacy criteria.

7. _____ pharmaceutical enterprises are stepping up efforts for high-quality innovations to propel drug research and development in pursuit of high-quality growth, according to experts and business executives.

8. The supervision _____ is committed to enforcing pharmaceutical standards and streamlining the drug approval process to ensure timely access to safe and effective medications.

9. The pharmaceutical regulatory agencies must _____ the entire drug production process, from initial development to market release, to ensure safety and efficacy standards are met.

10. In the safety assessment of drugs, it is crucial to _____ a comprehensive testing protocol that encompasses preclinical evaluations, clinical trials, and post-market surveillance to ensure the efficacy and minimize potential adverse effects.

11. The _____ of a drug's safety profile is crucial in determining its compliance with China's pharmaceutical standards, as it directly impacts patient safety and the regulatory landscape.

12. The regulatory authority will conduct a thorough _____ of the submitted data to ensure the safety and effectiveness of the drug.

13. The _____ of pharmaceutical products is subject to strict regulatory approval processes, which ensure that these products meet standards for safety and efficacy.

14. The World Health Organization classifies medications into various _____ based on their therapeutic uses and potential risks.

15. The efficacy of the novel therapeutic intervention was rigorously assessed through a comprehensive _____ of clinical trial data, which involved meta-analyses of outcomes from multiple patient cohorts.

II. Word Building

Study the Prefixes, Suffixes and Roots in the following grid, and then provide the corresponding word based on the given definition.

Prefixes	Meaning	Example
out-	"beyond" or "more than" (超越)	outweigh
com-	"together" or "with" (共同;与……一起)	compliance
over-	"above" or "on top of" (在上方)	oversee
Suffixes		
-ment	"the result or process of an action" (动作的结果或过程)	assessment
-tion	"the action, process, or state" (动作;过程;状态)	specification
Roots		
accord	"agreement" or "harmony" (一致;谐和)	accordance
spect	"to look" or "to observe" (看;观察)	inspection
import	"to bring or take into one's possession something that is foreign or not native" (进口或引入)	importation

1. the process in which something such as information, money, or goods passes from one person to another _____

2. to be out of agreement or to disagree with someone or something _____

3. to give someone more work or problems than they can deal with _____

4. a person you spend a lot of time with often because you are friends or because you are travelling together _____

5. to be greater in number than someone or something   _____

6. to think that someone has committed a crime or done something wrong

                                                                        _____

7. a person, country, or company that buys products from another country in order
   to sell them   _____

8. something that someone says or writes officially, or an action done to express an
   opinion   _____

9. too much of a drug taken or given at one time, either intentionally or by accident

                                                                        _____

10. a suggestion that something is good or suitable for a particular purpose or job

                                                                        _____

III. Structure & Function

Nominalization（名词化）is a grammatical process in which a verb or adjective is converted into a noun. This conversion changes the part of speech from a verb or adjective to a noun, which can be used as the subject or object of a sentence. For example:

Implement the new standards → *The implementation of the new standards*

Inspect manufacturing facilities → *Inspections of manufacturing facilities*

The drug manufacturing processes are monitored regularly to ensure that the companies comply with regulatory requirements.

→ *Regular monitoring of drug manufacturing processes is to ensure the companies' compliance with regulatory requirements.*

Here are pairs of sentences that convey the same meaning, with one sentence using nominalization and the other not:

1. *The development of the new drug took several years.* (nominalized structure)

   It took several years to develop the drug. (non-nominalized)

2. *The company is looking into the expansion of its market share.* (nominalized structure)

   The company is looking into expanding its market share. (non-nominalized)

3. *They discussed the allocation of resources at the meeting.* (nominalized structure)

    They discussed how to allocate resources at the meeting. (non-nominalized)

4. *She had a strong sense of responsibility towards her work.* (nominalized structure)

    She felt very responsible for her work. (non-nominalized)

In each pair, the first sentence uses a noun or noun phrase that has been created through nominalization, often by adding a suffix like -ment or -tion to a verb or adjective. The second sentence expresses the same idea without using nominalization, typically by using a verb or an infinitive construction.

Nominalization can make the sentence more concise and formal, and it can also make the sentence more complex and difficult to understand. In English, nominalization is a common grammatical phenomenon, and it is widely used in academic, legal and political writing.

Rewrite each of the following sentences, using a nominalized structure.

1. Implementing international pharmaceutical standards can help to improve access to medicines in developing countries.

   _____

   _____

2. Healthcare providers or pharmacists may perform routine testing on medications to ensure that they are still effective and safe for use.

   _____

   _____

3. It is crucial to monitor adverse reactions for patient safety during clinical trials.

   _____

   _____

4. When phase III trials are completed, it means the drug is ready for market approval.

5. To evaluate a drug's therapeutic efficacy, rigorous testing and analysis are often involved.

IV. Audio-visual Exercise

A. Listening Comprehension

Listen to a passage, which will be spoken only once. After you hear the passage, you must choose the best answer to each question from the four choices marked A, B, C, and D.

1. The passage is mainly about _____.
   A. preventing the spread of counterfeit medications
   B. distributing drugs in a safe and effective manner
   C. implementing international pharmaceutical standards
   D. protecting public health from substandard medications

2. International pharmaceutical standards are important in that they help to prevent _____.
   A. the damage to drug research integrity
   B. the production of counterfeit drugs
   C. the decrease in trust in medicines
   D. the increase in healthcare costs

3. International pharmaceutical standards also help to _____.
   A. reduce the risk of misuse of drugs
   B. protect the integrity of drug developers
   C. prevent the increase in healthcare costs
   D. ensure safe and effective distribution of drugs

4. By implementing international standards, developing countries can _____.
   A. improve access to medicines
   B. produce affordable medicines

C. drive down medication prices

D. reduce adverse drug reactions

5. By implementing international pharmaceutical standards, countries can do all of the following EXCEPT _____.

A. prevent the production of counterfeit drugs

B. make expertise and resources more attractive

C. distribute drugs with high levels of quality control

D. maintain the integrity of the pharmaceutical industry

B. Visual Comprehension

Watch a video clip three times and complete each of the following statements based on the video you have just watched.

1. Pfizer, the world's largest drug maker, agreed to pay $2.3 billion that is the largest fine in history, and agreed to plead guilty to charges it illegally marketed _____ for unapproved uses.

2. Dextra was approved by the FDA to treat pain from arthritis, but the drug giant Pfizer pitched doctors to prescribe the drug for things it was never approved for, called _____.

3. When off-label marketing like the case of Dextra occurs, patients' health and lives are put at risk and those who cause that risk must _____ _____.

4. The main whistle-blower, a former company sales representative, said in a statement that at Pfizer he was expected to increase profits at all costs, even when sales mean _____.

5. In the eight years, drug manufacturers have paid over $11 billion in penalties for everything from off-label promotions to _____.

V. Extended Reading

Read the following dialogue between Dr. Pharmed and students about the safety assessment and quality control of drugs, and complete each statement with a proper phrase or sentence given in the box.

Dr. Pharmed: Good morning, students of pharmacy. Today we will be discussing the safety assessment and quality control of drugs. Safety assessment is a critical process in drug development to ensure that medications are safe for use in humans. Quality control, on the other hand, is the process of ensuring that medications maintain their desired level of purity and potency throughout the manufacturing and distribution process.

Student 1: Can you explain how safety assessments are conducted?

Dr. Pharmed: Sure. Safety assessments typically involve several phases of testing, including preclinical studies in animals, followed by clinical trials in humans. Preclinical studies help researchers understand the effects of a drug on the body and identify potential side effects or toxicities. Clinical trials involve testing the drug on human subjects, usually in three phases — Phase I, II, and III. Phase I trials assess the drug's safety and dosage, Phase II trials evaluate its efficacy and further assess safety, and Phase III trials compare the drug to commonly used treatments in a larger population.

Student 2: What role does quality control play in ensuring drug safety?

Dr. Pharmed: Quality control is essential for maintaining the safety and efficacy of medications. It involves various processes, such as synthesis, formulation, manufacturing, packaging, storage, and distribution. These processes must be closely monitored to ensure that the final product is consistent in its composition, purity, and potency. Quality control also includes regular testing of drugs to detect any changes in their chemical structure or physical properties that could affect their safety or effectiveness.

Student 3: How do regulatory agencies oversee the safety and quality of drugs?

Dr. Pharmed: Regulatory agencies, such as the U.S. Food and Drug Administration (FDA) and the European Medicines Agency (EMA), play a crucial role in ensuring the safety and quality of drugs. They establish guidelines and regulations for drug development, manufacturing, and distribution. These agencies review the results of clinical trials and quality control data to determine whether a drug is safe and effective for use in humans. They also inspect pharmaceutical companies and their facilities to ensure compliance with good manufacturing practices (GMP).

Student 4: Are there any challenges in maintaining the safety and quality of drugs?

Dr. Pharmed: Yes, there are several challenges in maintaining the safety and quality of drugs. One challenge is the increasing complexity of drug development and manufacturing processes, which can lead to more opportunities for errors or contamination. Another challenge is the global nature of the pharmaceutical industry, which requires coordination between different countries and regulatory bodies. Additionally, emerging technologies, such as gene editing and personalized medicine, present new opportunities for improving drug safety and efficacy but also require careful evaluation to ensure they meet regulatory standards.

Student 5: How can pharmacists contribute to drug safety and quality control?

Dr. Pharmed: Pharmacists play a vital role in ensuring drug safety and quality control by providing accurate information to patients, monitoring their medication use, and reporting any adverse reactions or interactions. They also participate in quality control processes within pharmacies, such as verifying the authenticity of medications and checking expiration dates. Furthermore, pharmacists can advocate for better regulation and oversight of the pharmaceutical industry to improve overall drug safety and quality.

1. Assessment is a critical process in _____ by humans.
2. Phase III trials _____ on a larger scale.
3. To improve overall drug safety and quality, pharmacists can _____ .
4. Global nature of the pharmaceutical industry requires _____ .
5. Regulatory agencies set _____ and distribution of pharmaceuticals.

A. evaluate a drug's safety and effectiveness

B. compare the drug to commonly used treatment

C. drug development to guarantee their safe usage

D. advocate for better regulation and oversight of the industry

E. guidelines and regulations for the development, production

F. coordination between different countries and regulatory bodies

G. give patients correct details, keep track of their drug usage, and etc.

VI. Topics for Discussion and Essay-writing

1. Describe briefly the China's drug standard system.

2. How many stages are there in the clinical trials of drugs? What is the purpose of each stage?

3. Describe briefly the procedures for drug quality control.

Chapter VII

Future Trends in Drug Development and Application

7.1 The Globalization of Drug Development

The **globalization** of drug development refers to the process of pharmaceutical companies and research institutions **collaborating** and sharing resources on a global **scale** to **accelerate** the discovery, development, and commercialization of new drugs. With the advancements in technology and increasing global **connectivity**, the drug development process has become increasingly **globalized**.

Globalization of drug development enables pharmaceutical companies to **tap into** new pools of talent, ideas, and **resources** that may not be available within their local markets.

1. What is the concept of globalization of drug development?

2. What benefits does globalization of drug development bring to the drug companies?

globalization /ˌgləʊbələˈzeɪʃn/ *n*.	全球化;全球性
collaborate /kəˈlæbəreɪt/ *v*.	合作;协作;勾结
scale /skeɪl/ *n*.	规模;等级;标度
accelerate /əkˈseləreɪt/ *v*.	加速;加快
connectivity /ˌkɒnekˈtɪvɪtɪ/ *n*.	连接性;连通性
globalize /ˈgləʊbəlaɪz/ *v*.	(使)全球化
tap into	利用;开发
resource /ˈriːsɔːrs/ *n*.	资源;物力;财力

It can help speed up the drug development process by enabling companies to access **innovative** technologies, scientific expertise, and research resources from around the world. Additionally, global collaboration can help reduce costs by allowing companies to share expenses and resources, such as laboratory space and equipment.

One of the key drivers of globalization of drug development is the need for pharmaceutical companies to access new markets and customer bases. By collaborating with companies and research institutions in different regions, pharmaceutical companies can gain access to new cultural **insights**, market trends, and customer needs that can help them develop drugs that are more **relevant** and competitive in global markets.

3. What drives globalization of drug development?

Another important aspect of globalization of drug development is the ability to share risks and responsibilities. Drug development is a high-risk and high-cost process, with only a small percentage of drugs successfully making it to market. By collaborating with other companies and research institutions, pharmaceutical companies can spread the costs and risks associated with drug development, increasing their chances of success.

4. What is another benefit that drug companies gain from globalization of drug development?

Globalization of drug development also enables faster regulatory approvals and market access for drugs developed through collaboration. With the help of global regulatory agencies, drugs developed through collaboration can undergo multiple rounds of clinical trials and regulatory review in multiple regions **simultaneously**, reducing the

5. What else does drug developers gain from globalization of drug development?

---

innovative /ˈɪnəveɪtɪv/ *adj*.　　　　创新的;革新的;新颖的
insight /ˈɪnsaɪt/ *n*.　　　　　　　　洞察力;领悟;了解
relevant /ˈreləvənt/ *adj*.　　　　　相关的;相应的;适当的
simultaneously /ˌsɪməlˈteɪnɪəslɪ/ *adv*.　同时地;同步地;一齐

time and costs associated with developing drugs for multiple markets.

Overall, the globalization of drug development has opened up new opportunities for pharmaceutical companies and research institutions to collaborate, share resources, reduce costs, accelerate innovation, and access new markets. However, it also brings new challenges such as managing cultural differences, protecting intellectual property rights, and complying with different regulations in multiple markets.

6. What challenges do drug companies have to address with the globalization of drug development?

7.2 Trends Shaping the International Drug Market

The international drug market is constantly changing and being influenced by various trends. Here are some of the main trends shaping the market today:

Diversification of the market: One of the key trends shaping the international drug market is diversification of the market, which means that drugs are not only sold for medicinal purposes, but also for **cosmetic** and **nutraceutical** uses. This trend has been growing in recent years, as more people pay attention to health and beauty and seek out new ways to maintain their health and appearance. The cosmetics and nutraceuticals market is expected to expand significantly in the coming years, providing drug companies with new opportunities to develop innovative products that meet consumer demand.

1. What is meant by diversification of the market?

2. What is the reason for the growing trend of diversification of the market?

---

diversification /daɪˌvɜːsɪfɪˈkeɪʃn/ *n.*   多样化;变化;多种经营
cosmetic /kɒzˈmetɪks/ *n./adj.*   美容品(的);化妆品(的)
nutraceutical /ˈnuːtrəˈsuːtɪkəl/ *n./adj.*   营养食品(的);保健食品(的)

Increasing role of innovation and technology: Another important trend is the increasing role of innovation and technology in driving the development of the drug market. With the continuous advancement of science and technology, the costs of drug research and development have been decreasing, while the speed of innovation has been increasing. This trend has led to more innovative drugs that can be brought to the market in a shorter period of time. In addition, technology has also been playing a crucial role in drug production processes, ensuring higher quality and more **cost-effective** production. Drug companies are using advanced manufacturing technologies, such as continuous manu-facturing and **microfluidics**, to improve production efficiency and reduce costs.

Digitalization and **e-commerce**: Digitalization and e-commerce are revolutionizing the way drugs are sold and marketed. Online sales **channels** provide drug companies with new opportunities to reach customers directly and expand their customer base. Drug companies are using digital marketing **strategies**, such as social media advertising and **influencer** marketing, to promote their products and build brand awareness. In addition, online pharmacies are becoming more popular, providing consumers with convenient access to drugs while ensuring safety and quality control.

3. *What is another important trend shaping the drug market?*

4. *What results from the continuous advancement of science and technology?*

5. *How are digitalization and e-commerce revolutionizing the way drugs are sold and marketed?*

---

cost-effective /ˌkɒst ɪˈfektɪv/ *adj.*　　有成本效益的；划算的
microfluidics /maɪkrəʊfluˈɪdɪks/ *n.*　　微流体
digitalization /ˌdɪdʒətəlaɪˈzeɪʃən/ *n.*　　数字化
e-commerce /iːˈkɒmɜːs/ *n.*　　电子商务
channel /ˈtʃænl/ *n.*　　渠道；途径；门路
strategy /ˈstrætədʒɪ/ *n.*　　战略；策略；部署
influencer /ˈɪnfluənsər/ *n.*　　有影响的人（或事物）

Personalized medicine and **precision** health: Personalized medicine and precision health are trends that are revolutionizing the way drugs are developed and prescribed. Drug companies are using advanced genetic testing and other technologies to develop personalized drug regimens that are tailored to individual patients' needs and respond to their specific genetic **traits**. This approach can help to improve treatment outcomes and reduce side effects while ensuring that drugs are used more cost-effectively. In addition, precision health **interventions**, such as targeted drug delivery and wearable health devices, are being developed to provide better care for patients while reducing the burden on healthcare systems.

6. How are personalized medicine and precision health revolutionizing the way drugs are developed and prescribed?

Impact of the internet on the drug market: The internet has had a significant impact on the drug market. It has provided easier access to information about drugs and their uses, while also allowing for direct sales of drugs online. This trend has presented both opportunities and challenges for drug companies, as it provides new channels for sales and marketing but also raises issues related to regulations and safety concerns. The ease of online shopping for drugs has made it more convenient for consumers to **purchase** medication, but it has also opened up new **avenues** for illegal activities, such as counterfeiting and **diversion** of drugs. Therefore, drug companies need to

7. How does the internet impact the drug market?

---

precision /prɪˈsɪʒn/ *n*.　　　　　　精确;精密
trait /treɪt/ *n*.　　　　　　　　　　特点;特征;特性
intervention /ˌɪntərˈvenʃn/ *n*.　　　介入;干预;干涉
purchase /ˈpɜːrtʃəs/ *v*.　　　　　　购买;采购
avenue /ˈævənuː/ *n*.　　　　　　　途径;方法;林荫道
diversion /daɪˈvɜːrʒn/ *n*.　　　　　转向;转移;临时绕行路

be **proactive** in addressing these challenges while taking advantage of the opportunities presented by the internet.

Language Practice

I. Vocabulary Work

Complete each of the following sentences with a suitable word or expression given below.

collaborate	resource	cost-effective	trait
scale	innovative	digitalization	intervention
accelerate	insight	channel	purchase
connectivity	relevant	strategy	diversion
tap into	simultaneously	influencer	proactive

1. To accelerate the globalization of drug development, pharmaceutical companies are _____ with research institutions and governments to share resources and expertise.
2. To stay ahead in the competitive global market, pharmaceutical companies must adopt a _____ approach to drug development by anticipating and addressing regional regulatory requirements early on in the process.
3. In recent years, the use of artificial intelligence and machine learning has become more _____ in the global drug development process, reducing the time and resources needed for preclinical research.
4. The globalization of drug development has provided researchers with new _____ into the genetic and environmental factors that contribute to disease.
5. The increased _____ between research institutions and pharmaceutical companies across different regions has facilitated the sharing of knowledge and resources in the global drug development process.
6. Pharmaceutical companies are developing new _____ to accelerate drug

---

proactive /ˌprəʊˈæktɪv/ *adj.*　　　　　　积极的；主动的；主动出击的

development in response to the growing demand for innovative treatments in a globalized market.

7. Research institutions are adopting collaborative strategies to share knowledge and resources, improving the efficiency and effectiveness of drug development on a global _____ .

8. The globalization of drug development has led to an increase in the _____ of pharmaceuticals, as drugs intended for one market are sold in another without authorization.

9. The globalization of drug development has led to the emergence of _____ new treatments that address the unique health needs of patients in different regions.

10. Governments and international organizations are implementing _____ to support the development and distribution of drugs in underserved regions, reducing health disparities on a global scale.

11. Pharmaceutical companies are _____ emerging markets to expand their customer base and increase revenue in a globalized economy.

12. The globalization of drug development has made it essential for researchers to consider the cultural and social factors that are _____ to the health needs of diverse populations.

13. The globalization of drug development has _____ the pace of innovation, enabling pharmaceutical companies to bring new treatments to market more quickly than ever before.

14. By analyzing data from clinical trials conducted in different regions _____ , researchers can gain insights into the effectiveness and safety of drugs across diverse populations.

15. By studying the genetic _____ of patients in different regions, pharmaceutical companies can develop drugs that are tailored to the unique needs of each population.

II. Word Building

Study the Prefixes, Suffixes and Roots in the following grid, and then provide the corresponding word based on the given definition.

Prefixes	Meaning	Example
co-	"together" or "in partnership"（共同；合作）	collaborate
pro-	"in favor of" or "supporting"（赞成；支持）	proactive
Suffixes		
-er	"someone who does something"（做……的人）	influencer
-ity	"a quality or state"（品质或状态）	connectivity
Roots		
labor	"work" or "toil"（工作；苦干）	collaborate
celer	"swift" or "quick"（迅速；快）	accelerate
digit	"a number or a numerical figure"（数目；数字）	digitalization
connect	"to join" or "to attach"（连接）	connectivity

1. to work together or collaborate with someone or something, emphasizing the joint effort and cooperation among individuals or groups　_____

2. taking positive action or measures to anticipate and address future situations or problems　_____

3. someone who writes books, articles, or other written materials　_____

4. the state or quality of being equal or fair　_____

5. the state or quality of being real or actual　_____

6. a person who works with their hands, typically doing heavy or unskilled work

　_____

7. involving hard or tiring work　_____

8. relating to or using digits or the numerical values that represent information in a computer or similar device　_____

9. to move quickly or increase the speed of something　_____

10. the state of being connected; a relationship in which a person or thing is linked or associated with something else　_____

III. Structure & Function

The "by + -ing phrase" structure is used to express the means or method by which something is accomplished. It indicates how an action is performed or how a result is achieved. For example：

Global collaboration can help reduce costs <u>by allowing companies to share expenses and resources</u>, such as laboratory space and equipment.

It can help speed up the drug development process <u>by enabling companies to access innovative technologies, scientific expertise, and research resources from around the world</u>.

<u>By collaborating with companies and research institutions in different regions</u>, pharmaceutical companies can gain access to new cultural insights, market trends, and customer needs

Apart from the "by + -ing phrase", there are several other prepositional phrases or structures that can be used to express the means or method by which something is accomplished. Here are a few examples:

1. Through + noun/pronoun: This phrase is used to describe the agency or intermediary through which something is achieved. For example:

With the help of global regulatory agencies, drugs developed <u>through collaboration</u> can undergo multiple rounds of clinical trials and regulatory review in multiple regions simultaneously.

2. By means of + noun/gerund: This phrase indicates the method or strategy employed to achieve a goal. For example:

The company is developing a new drug to treat Alzheimer's disease <u>by means of a novel delivery system</u>.

3. With + noun/pronoun: This structure is used to indicate the tool, object, or resource that is used to perform an action. For example:

<u>With the help of modern genetic engineering techniques</u>, researchers are able to create new drugs with fewer side effects.

4. Using + noun/gerund: This structure is similar to "with + noun/pronoun" and specifies the tool, method, or resource employed for an action. For example:

The company has developed a new method for manufacturing drugs, <u>using sustainable and environmentally friendly processes</u>.

Each of these phrases and structure provides different nuances about how something is accomplished, and their use depends on the context and the specific details being emphasized in the sentence.

Translate the following sentences, using in each an expression given in parentheses.

1. 在计算机建模的帮助下,药物化学家能够利用虚拟筛选技术设计新药。(using+noun/gerund)

   _____

   _____

2. 该公司结合传统中医药与现代技术,开发出了独特的慢性疼痛治疗方法。(by+-ing phrase)

   _____

   _____

3. 通过开发新药,医疗专业人员能够治疗以前无法治疗的疾病,并延长患者的生命。(through+noun/pronoun)

   _____

   _____

4. 在现代技术的帮助下,药物开发人员能够创造出更有效、更安全的药物,并减少副作用。(with+noun/pronoun)

   _____

   _____

5. 该公司利用高通量筛选和计算建模的结合,并通过虚拟现实技术来识别潜在的药物候选物。(by means of+noun/gerund)

   _____

   _____

IV. Audio-visual Exercise

A. Listening Comprehension

Listen to a passage, which will be spoken only once. After you hear the passage, you must choose the best answer to each question from the four choices marked A, B, C, and D.

1. The passage is mainly about _____ .

    A. the globalization of drug development

    B. ethical considerations related to drug research

    C. increased competition among drug developers

    D. technological advancements in drug development

2. Faced with increased competition, companies are looking for ways to _____ .

    A. produce affordable medicines

    B. share their knowledge and resources

    C. maintain the integrity of drug research

    D. accelerate the drug development process

3. Which of the following is mentioned as an advance in technology for researchers to collaborate across borders?

    A. Bioinformatics.   B. Teleconferencing.

    C. Genetic engineering.   D. Artificial intelligence.

4. Companies are under increasing pressure to demonstrate that their products are safe and effective because of _____ .

    A. the more complex regulatory environment

    B. the increasingly competitive environment

    C. the effective collaboration between researchers

    D. the fast-growing demand for affordable medicines

5. Which of the following is NOT mentioned as a risk associated the globalization of drug development?

    A. Ethical concerns.   B. Cultural differences.

    C. Stringent regulations.   D. Intellectual property disputes.

B. Visual Comprehension

Watch a video three times and complete each of the following statements based on the video you have just watched.

1. Anne Doudna and her collaborator Emmanuelle Charpentier won the Nobel for their 2012 work on a scientific breakthrough: _____
_____ known as CRISPR.

2. CRISPR is an acronym that stands for Clustered, _____ ,
Palindromic, and Repeats.

3. Since Doudna published her paper in 2012, a lot has been going on in _____

_____ using CRISPR techniques.

4. About 7,000 human diseases are caused by gene mutations, including sickle cell disease, a blood disorder that brings debilitating pain, _____

_____ .

5. Victoria Gray, a Mississippi mother of four who became the first American to be treated with CRISPR-fixed genes. In the years since the experimental treatment, she _____ .

V. Extended Reading

Read the following dialogue between Dr. Pharmed and students about the trends that are shaping the international drug market, and complete the dialogue with a suitable phrase or sentence from the grid.

Dr. Pharmed: Hi, everybody. Have you heard about the trends that are shaping the international drug market?

Student 1: No, I haven't. What are those trends?

Dr. Pharmed: Well, one of them is the growing importance of emerging drug markets like China, India, and Brazil. With their large populations and growing middle class, these countries are expected ___1___ .

Student 2: That's interesting. What else?

Dr. Pharmed: Another trend is the shift towards personalized medicine. Advances in genomics, proteomics, and other areas of biotechnology are enabling researchers to develop more targeted and personalized treatments for patients. This trend is expected ___2___ .

Student 3: That sounds promising. What about digital transformation in the pharmaceutical industry?

Dr. Pharmed: Yes, definitely. The COVID-19 pandemic has accelerated the digital transformation of the pharmaceutical industry, with many companies investing in technologies such as telemedicine, e-prescriptions, and digital therapeutics. This trend is expected to continue, with companies using technology ___3___ .

Student 4: It's interesting to see how different trends are shaping the international drug market. What about antimicrobial resistance?

Dr. Pharmed: Yes, that's a significant threat to public health worldwide. As a result, there is increased interest in developing new antimicrobial agents and improving existing ones to combat AMR. This trend is expected to shape the international drug market, with companies working __4__ and governments implementing policies to address drug affordability.

Student 5: It's clear that the international drug market is evolving rapidly, with various factors driving these trends. Thanks for sharing this information with us!

Dr. Pharmed: You're welcome! It's always important __5__.

_____ 1	A. to develop more affordable treatments
_____ 2	B. to be proactive in addressing the challenges
_____ 3	C. to become major players in the global drug market
_____ 4	D. to stay informed about these changes in the industry
_____ 5	E. to shape the development and approval of new drugs in the future
	F. to improve patient outcomes, increase efficiency, and reduce costs
	G. to keep track of the latest advances in drug research and development

VI. Topics for Discussion and Essay-writing

1. What opportunities does the globalization of drug development bring to pharmaceutical companies?

2. What challenges does the globalization of drug development bring to pharmaceutical companies?

3. How does the Internet impact the global drug market?

7.3   Artificial Intelligence & the Development of New Drugs

Artificial intelligence (AI) has the potential to revolutionize the development of new drugs by accelerating and **streamlining** the process, reducing costs, and improving success rates.

One of the key areas where AI is being applied in drug development is in the identification and **validation** of drug targets. Traditional drug discovery processes often involve **extensive** screening of potential targets through laboratory experiments, which is **time-consuming** and costly. With AI, however, it is possible to use computer-aided **docking simulations** to **predict** how potential drugs will **interact** with their target proteins, greatly reducing the need for **laborious** laboratory experiments.

Another area where AI is making an impact in drug development is in the **prediction** and optimization of drug candidates' properties. Drug candidates need to possess certain chemical and biological properties to be effective against a particular disease, and traditional drug design

1. What is one key area where AI is being applied in drug development?

2. What shortcomings are mentioned about traditional drug processes?

3. What are other advantages of AI in drug development compared with traditional drug design methods?

streamline /ˈstriːmlaɪn/ v.　使(过程等)精简;效率更高
validation /ˌvælɪˈdeɪʃn/ n.　确证;确认;证明……有价值
extensive /ɪkˈstensɪv/ adj.　广泛的;全面的
time-consuming /ˈtaɪm kənsuːmɪŋ/ adj.　耗时的;费时的
docking /ˈdɒkɪŋ/ n.　对接;船停靠码头
simulation /ˌsɪmjʊˈleɪʃn/ n.　模仿;模拟;仿真品
predict /prɪˈdɪkt/ v.　预言;预测;预告
interact /ˌɪntərˈækt/ v.　相互作用;交流;互动
laborious /ləˈbɔːrɪəs/ adj.　耗时费力的;辛苦的;艰难的
prediction /prɪˈdɪkʃn/ n.　预测;预报;预言

methods often involve extensive testing and **iterative** experiments to achieve the desired properties. By contrast, AI algorithms can use machine learning techniques to analyze vast amounts of data on drug candidates' properties to predict their effectiveness and safety in humans, optimizing their design before preclinical trials even begin.

AI can also support decision-making during the clinical trials phase of drug development. For example, AI algorithms can analyze medical records and electronic health data to identify suitable patients for **enrollment** in trials, and can also analyze data collected during trials to predict trial outcomes and inform decision-making on whether to continue, modify, or **terminate** trials.

4. How can AI support decision-making during the clinical trials of drug development?

Overall, artificial intelligence has the potential to **transform** drug development by greatly accelerating the process, reducing costs, and improving the quality and success rate of drugs. It represents a new **frontier** in the field of pharmaceutical research and development that has the potential to bring about a revolution in patient care.

5. What is the significance of AI being applied in drug development?

---

iterative /ˈɪtəˌreɪtɪv/ *adj*.	重复的；反复的；迭代的
enrollment /enˈrəʊlmənt/ *n*.	登记；注册
terminate /ˈtɜːrmɪneɪt/ *v*.	(使)终止；(使)结束
transform /trænsˈfɔːrm/ *v*.	转换；改变；改造
frontier /frʌnˈtɪə(r)/ *n*.	前沿；新领域；边界

7.4   Application of Biopharmaceutical Technologies

Biopharmaceutical technologies have the potential to significantly impact drug development and improve patient outcomes. Here are some of the most **promising** biopharmaceutical technologies for drug development:

Gene **editing**: Gene editing technologies such as **CRISPR**-Cas9 can be used to **edit** genes responsible for certain diseases, potentially leading to the development of new drugs.

Cell-based therapies: Cell-based therapies involve using cells or **tissues** from a patient's own body to create a drug that is tailored to their specific needs. This approach has the potential to reduce side effects and improve efficacy compared to traditional drug therapies.

Personalized medicine: Advances in **genomics** and other technologies are allowing for the creation of personalized medicine, where treatments are tailored to an individual's genetic **makeup**. This can lead to more effective and targeted treatments.

1. What role will biopharmaceutical technologies play in drug development?

2. What is said about cell-based therapies compared with traditional drug therapies?

biopharmaceutical /baɪnfɑːməˈsjuːtɪkl/ *adj.*　　生物制药学
promising /ˈprɒmɪsɪŋ/ *adj.*　　很有前途的;前景很好的
editing /ˈedɪtɪŋ/ *n.*　　编辑;剪辑
CRISPR /ˈkrɪspər/ *abbr.*　　成簇规则间隔短回文重复序列 (Clustered Regularly Interspaced Short Palindromic Repeats)
edit /ˈedɪt/ *v.*　　编辑;剪辑;主编
tissue /ˈtɪʃuː/ *n.*　　组织;薄纸;面巾纸
genomics /dʒəˈnɒmɪks/ *n.*　　基因组学
makeup /ˈmeɪˌkʌp/ *n.*　　组成成分;构成;构造

Artificial intelligence: AI can be used to analyze large amounts of data and identify potential drug candidates more quickly and accurately than traditional methods.

Nanotechnology: Nanotechnology involves **manipulating** materials on a **molecular** scale, which could lead to the development of new drugs with improved efficacy and reduced side effects.

3. How is nanotechnology related to drug development?

Overall, these biopharmaceutical technologies have the potential to revolutionize drug development by increasing efficiency, reducing costs, and improving outcomes for patients. However, there are also challenges associated with implementing these technologies, such as regulatory **barriers** and ethical concerns around the use of gene editing and other advanced techniques in drug development.

4. What are some challenges associated with implementing those technologies?

7.5 Personalized Medicine & Drug Development

Personalized medicine refers to the tailoring of medical treatment to the specific **characteristics** of each individual patient, taking into account their genetic background, lifestyle, environment, and other factors. In drug development, personalized medicine has the potential to transform the way drugs are designed and prescribed, leading to more targeted and effective treatment options

1. What is the concept of personalized medicine?

---

nanotechnology /ˌnænəʊtekˈnɒlədʒɪ/ n.　　纳米技术
manipulate /məˈnɪpjʊleɪt/ v.　　操作;处理;控制
molecular /məˈlekjələr/ adj.　　分子的;与分子有关的
barrier /ˈbærɪər/ n.　　障碍;壁垒;阻碍
characteristic /ˌkærəktəˈrɪstɪk/ adj.　　明显的;典型的;独特的

for patients.

One aspect of personalized medicine in drug development is the use of genetic testing to identify patients who may respond better to a particular drug based on their genetic profile. This **approach** can help drug companies develop drugs that are more likely to work in specific patient populations, reducing the number of side effects and improving efficacy.

2. *What is used in personalized medicine in drug development?*

Another aspect of personalized medicine is the use of individualized drug **regimens**, which are designed based on a patient's specific characteristics and needs. These drug regimens may involve targeted drugs that are designed to act on specific biological markers or pathways involved in a particular disease, as well as drugs that are tailored to individual patients' response and **tolerance** levels.

3. *Why are individualized drug regimens used in personalized medicine?*

In addition, personalized medicine also includes the use of precision health interventions, such as wearable health devices and mobile health apps, that can monitor a patient's health **status** and medication use in **real-time**. This information can help doctors adjust drug dosage or **switch** to alternative drugs in a timely manner, ensuring optimal treatment for patients.

4. *What is the use of wearable health devices in personalized medicine?*

Overall, personalized medicine has the potential to improve drug development and delivery by better tailoring treatment options to the needs of individual patients. It

5. *What are the overall advantages of personalized medicine?*

---

approach /əˈprəʊtʃ/ n.　　　　路径；途径；方法；方式
regimen /ˈredʒɪmən/ n.　　　　养生法；养生之道；生活规则
tolerance /ˈtɒlərəns/ n.　　　　忍耐(力)；忍受(力)；耐药性
status /ˈsteɪtəs/ n.　　　　　　地位；状态；情形
real-time　　　　　　　　　　即时处理的；实时的
switch /swɪtʃ/ v.　　　　　　　转换；改变；转变

can help doctors personalize their prescribing decisions, improve patient outcomes, and reduce healthcare costs associated with ineffective or unnecessary treatment.

Language Practice

I. Vocabulary Work

Complete each of the following sentences with a suitable word or expression given below.

streamline	interact	transform	barrier
validation	laborious	frontier	characteristic
extensive	prediction	promising	approach
simulation	iterative	edit	regimen
enrollment	terminate	manipulate	tolerance

1. The AI-driven platform is _____ the drug discovery process by rapidly analyzing vast datasets to identify potential drug candidates with unprecedented speed and accuracy.

2. Through advanced computational _____, AI is enabling the prediction of drug interactions at a molecular level, which is crucial for designing safer and more effective medications.

3. The AI-driven _____ to drug discovery is shifting the focus from trial-and-error to data-driven insights, significantly increasing the success rate of clinical trials.

4. The ability of AI to _____ with large-scale molecular databases allows researchers to identify new drug candidates by simulating their interactions with biological targets.

5. The _____ use of AI in drug development has led to a significant acceleration in the identification and optimization of lead compounds, reducing the time from discovery to market.

6. The biopharmaceutical company decided to _____ the clinical trial early after AI analysis indicated that the drug was unlikely to achieve its therapeutic goals.

7. The biopharmaceutical industry is constantly innovating to develop drugs with

new _____ , such as improved stability and reduced immuno-genicity, to enhance patient outcomes.

8. Biopharmaceutical researchers are adept at _____ genes to produce recombinant proteins, which are then used to develop targeted therapies for various diseases.

9. Researchers are excited about the _____ potential of CRISPR technology in biopharmaceuticals, as it offers a precise method for editing genes to treat genetic disorders.

10. The successful _____ of a diagnostic test for a specific genetic mutation is a significant milestone in the field of personalized medicine, as it enables more accurate patient stratification and treatment planning.

11. The ethical implications of gene editing in personalized medicine are a topic of intense debate, as the ability to _____ human DNA raises questions about the long-term consequences and societal impact.

12. The _____ of patients into a personalized medicine clinical trial is a critical step, as it ensures that each participant's unique genetic profile is considered in the treatment plan.

13. The development of personalized treatment plans in oncology takes into account the patient's _____ to specific chemotherapy drugs, ensuring that the therapy is both effective and tolerable.

14. The cost of advanced genetic testing can be a _____ for many patients seeking personalized medicine, potentially limiting access to treatments tailored to their genetic makeup.

15. The development of a personalized medication _____ for managing chronic conditions is a key area of growth in the field of personalized medicine, offering hope for more effective patient care.

II. Word Building

Study the Prefixes, Suffixes and Roots in the following grid, and then provide the corresponding word based on the given definition.

Prefixes	Meaning	Example
trans-	"across," "over," "through," or "beyond"（穿越,超越）	transform
pre-	"before" or "ahead of"（在……前或先于……）	prediction
nano-	"dwarf" or "one billionth"（矮小或十亿分之一）	nanotechnology
Suffixes		
-ance	"an action or state"（动作或状态）	tolerance
Roots		
termin	"end" or "finish"（终止;结束）	terminate
valid	"strong, firm, healthy, or having legal force"（强;牢;有法律效力的）	validation
form	"shape" or "structure"（形状;结构）	transform
dict	"speak or say"（讲;说）	predict

1. the act of dictating or the practice of writing down spoken words as they are spoken _____

2. to stop something from happening before it occurs _____

3. having an abnormal or irregular shape _____

4. not valid or legally binding; lacking legal force or effect _____

5. the act of ending or bringing something to a close _____

6. the quality of being important or meaningful _____

7. the act of conforming to rules, standards, or requests _____

8. to transfer a plant or organ from one place to another, especially for medical purposes _____

9. the application of nanotechnology in the medical field, such as drug delivery systems at the nanoscale _____

10. something done to avoid danger or problems before they happen _____

III. Structure & Function

Impersonal sentence structures with a non-personal subject "It" are often used in scientific, technical, or objective writing, where the focus is on general truths or facts rather than on personal experiences or specific events. For example:

It is important to eat a balanced diet.

It is recommended that you drink plenty of water during exercise.

It is essential that cutting-edge technologies are used in drug development to ensure the safety and efficacy of new drugs.

It happens that technologies in drug development are now able to personalize treatment for individual patients, allowing for the tailoring of drugs based on their unique genetic and environmental factors.

"There is …" and "There are …" are also impersonal sentence structures, which are used to introduce a subject or subjects that are not directly involved in any action or thought expressed in the sentence. For example:

There is a need for further research and development in biopharmaceutical technologies to improve the safety, efficacy, and cost-effectiveness of these drugs.

There are also challenges associated with implementing these technologies, such as regulatory barriers and ethical concerns around the use of gene editing.

Overall, these sentence structures are often used in impersonal or objective contexts, such as news articles, scientific reports, or official documents. They promote objectivity, facilitate the explanation of complex ideas or processes and avoid the potential subjectivity that can arise when referring to personal thoughts or actions.

Translate the following sentences, using in each an impersonal sentence structure.

1. 在批准新药用于患者之前,进行严格的临床试验以确保其安全性和有效性是至关重要的。

   _____

   _____

2. 预计技术进步将继续在新药开发中发挥重要作用,为患者带来更有效、更安全的治疗选择。

   _____

   _____

3. 有各种新技术可供企业使用来提高运营效率和增加效益,例如人工智能、机器学习和机器人技术。

4. 新技术在药物开发中的应用显著提高了在分子水平上对疾病的理解,使得能够识别新的药物治疗靶点,并开发出更有效、更安全的药物。

5. 人们对将生物制药技术应用于个性化医学的兴趣不断增长,因为个性化医学旨在根据患者独特的遗传和环境因素为他们量身定制治疗方案。

IV. Audio-visual Exercise

A. Listening Comprehension

Listen to a passage, which will be spoken only once. After you hear the passage, you must choose the best answer to each question from the four choices marked A, B, C, and D.

1. It is mentioned that AI has the potential to do all of the following EXCEPT _____.

    A. make predictions about drug efficacy

    B. reduce the time and cost of R & D

    C. analyze large amounts of data

    D. select suitable candidates

2. Machine learning algorithms can help researchers to focus on _____.

    A. identifying the most promising leads

    B. analyzing vast amounts of data

    C. predicting different compounds

    D. conducting genetic studies

3. AI can identify potential _____ much faster than traditional methods.

    A. cost and risks

    B. drug candidates

    C. chemical databases

    D. genomes and proteins

4. How can AI improve the efficiency of clinical trials?

   A. By improving product quality.

   B. By optimizing the time for clinical trials.

   C. By identifying suitable patients for trials.

   D. By allowing doctors to take corrective action.

5. The passage mainly discusses AI's potential to _____ .

   A. revolutionize drug research and development

   B. bring new pharmaceuticals to market

   C. improve the efficiency of clinical trials

   D. optimize manufacturing processes

B. Visual Comprehension

Watch a video clip three times and complete each of the following statements based on the video you have just watched.

1. Jack was born with retinitis pigmentosa, a _____ causing blindness, which will probably cause his sight loss by the time he's 20 or 30 years old.

2. Jack was the first person in the United States to receive an FDA approved gene therapy. A new drug Luxturna was injected into his eye to _____

   _____ .

3. Jack's vision improved dramatically, but _____

   is $850,000.

4. An independent watchdog group which studies drug costs said Luxturna is overpriced, and arrived at a figure of approximately $400,000 to $450,000 as

   a _____ .

5. The gene therapy is really effective and really expensive, but for families like Jack, the science _____ .

V. Extended Reading

Read the following dialogue between Dr. Pharmed and students about biopharmaceutical technologies, and choose the best answer to each question according to the dialogue.

Dr. Pharmed: Hello, everyone! Today we're going to talk about biopharmaceutical technologies. These are technologies that use living organisms to produce drugs. They are revolutionizing the way we develop and produce drugs.

Student 1: That sounds interesting. What are some examples of biopharmaceutical technologies?

Dr. Pharmed: One example is monoclonal antibodies. These are proteins produced by cloned cells that bind to specific targets in the body, such as cancer cells. Another example is gene therapy, which involves the delivery of genes to cells to treat genetic diseases or infections.

Student 2: How do these technologies work?

Dr. Pharmed: In the case of monoclonal antibodies, we take a mouse with a cancer and inject it with a virus that will make the mouse produce human antibodies against the cancer. We then clone the cells that produce these antibodies and use them to make the drug. For gene therapy, we deliver the correct gene to replace the faulty gene that causes the disease.

Student 3: Are these technologies safe?

Dr. Pharmed: Safety is always a concern when it comes to drugs, but biopharmaceutical technologies have been shown to be effective and safe in many cases. However, like any new technology, we need to continue to monitor their safety and efficacy carefully.

Student 4: What are the benefits of these technologies?

Dr. Pharmed: The benefits are many. One of the main benefits is that these technologies allow us to produce drugs in large quantities and with high purity, which reduces the risk of side effects. Additionally, these technologies can be used to develop drugs that are difficult to produce using traditional methods, such as proteins or peptides.

Student 5: Are there any downsides to these technologies?

Dr. Pharmed: Yes, there are some downsides. One of the main issues is the cost of developing and producing drugs using biopharmaceutical technologies. It can be very expensive and may limit access to these drugs for some patients. Additionally, like any new technology, there can be unforeseen risks or side effects that we need to be aware of.

Student 6: What's the future of biopharmaceutical technologies?

Dr. Pharmed: The future looks very promising for biopharmaceutical technologies. With advances in technology and research, we expect to see more drugs developed using these methods in the future. Additionally, we may see more personalized medicine using these technologies, where drugs are tailored to individual patients based on their unique biology.

1. Which of the following is NOT an example of biopharmaceutical technology?

   A. Radiotherapy.   B. Antiviral therapy.

   C. Gene therapy.   D. Cell therapy.

2. All of the following are concerned with monoclonal antibodies EXCEPT _____.

   A. use the cells with antibodies to make a drug

   B. deliver the correct gene to replace the faulty gene

   C. take a mouse with a cancer and inject it with a virus

   D. make the mouse produce human antibodies against the cancer

3. Which of the following is NOT mentioned as a benefit of biopharmaceutical technologies?

   A. Produce drugs in large quantities and with high purity.

   B. Develop drugs difficult to produce such as proteins.

   C. Replace the traditional manufacturing methods.

   D. Use living organisms to produce drugs.

4. Downsides of using biopharmaceutical technologies to produce drugs include _____.

   A. expensive costs

   B. unforeseen risks

   C. potential side effects

   D. all of the above mentioned

5. Which of the following shows a promising future for biopharmaceutical technologies?

    A. More personalized medicine using these technologies.

    B. More drugs developed using non-traditional methods.

    C. More advances in drug research and development.

    D. More advances in cancer treatment based on DNA.

VI. Topics for Discussion and Essay-writing

1. Why is there a trend for AI to be increasingly used in drug research and development?

2. What are potential challenges associated with implementing AI in drug development?

3. How will biopharmaceutical technology significantly impact drug development and improve patient outcomes in the future?

Chapter VIII

Pharmacy Education and Career Development

8.1 Pharmacy Education at Multilevels

Pharmacy education is a multi-leveled program that typically includes the following levels:

Bachelor of Science in Pharmacy (BSP): This is the entry-level degree for pharmacy students, and it typically takes four years to complete. During this time, students will learn about basic pharmacology, drug interactions, and other **foundational** topics in pharmacy.

1. What is the entry-level degree for pharmacy students?

Doctor of Pharmacy (PharmD) or Doctor of **Osteopathic** Medicine (ODM): This advanced degree program requires an additional two to three years of **coursework** beyond the BSP. Students who **pursue** this degree will typically specialize in a particular area

2. In what area will students pursue the degree of Doctor of Pharmacy?

---

pharmacy /ˈfɑːrməsɪ/ n.　　　　　　药学;药剂学;药房;制药业
bachelor /ˈbætʃələr/ n.　　　　　　学士;单身汉
foundational /faʊnˈdeɪʃənəl/ adj.　　基本的;基础的
osteopathic /ˌɒstɪrˈpæθɪk/ adj.　　　整骨疗法的
coursework /ˈkɔːswɜːk/ n.　　　　　(计入最终成绩的)课程作业
pursue /pərˈsuː/ v.　　　　　　　　寻求;追求;继续

of pharmacy, such as clinical pharmacy or research pharmacy.

Master of Science in Pharmacy (MSP): This is an advanced degree program that can be pursued by those who already have a PharmD or BSP. MSP programs typically focus on specialized areas of pharmacy, such as pharmaceutical research or clinical practice management.

Postdoctoral Certificate Program: This is a postgraduate certificate program that can be pursued by individuals who already have a PharmD or BSP. These programs typically last one to two years and provide advanced training in a specific area of pharmacy, such as clinical pharmacy or pharmacology.

3. *Who may pursue Postdoctoral Certificate Programs?*

In addition to these degrees, many colleges and universities offer various pharmacy programs and **certifications**, such as the American **Pharmacist** Association's Certified Pharmacy Technician (CPHT) certification or the National Association of Boards of Pharmacy's **Certified** Health Education Specialist (CHES) certification. These programs can help individuals advance their careers and gain specialized knowledge in different areas of pharmacy.

4. *What is the use of other pharmacy programs such as CHES?*

---

postdoctoral /ˌpəʊstˈdɒktərəl/ *adj.*　　博士后的
certification /ˌsɜːrtɪfɪˈkeɪʃn/ *n.*　　课程结业证书；证明；鉴定
pharmacist /ˈfɑːməsɪst/ *n.*　　药剂师
certify /ˈsɜːrtɪfaɪ/ *v.*　　(出具)证明；给……颁发结业证书

8. 2   Career Paths Available to Graduates of Pharmacy

Pharmacy graduates can pursue a variety of career paths, including:

Pharmacist: This is the most common career path for pharmacy graduates. Pharmacists provide patient care and advice on **medication** use, manage **prescription** medications, and dispense over-the-counter medications. To become a pharmacist, individuals must meet certain requirements and pass pharmacist licensing examinations, for example, individuals in the U. S. must complete a PharmD degree program and pass the North American Pharmacist Licensing Examination (NAPLEX).

1. What is the most common career path for pharmacy graduates?

Medical Science Researcher: Pharmacy graduates with advanced degrees, such as PharmD or MSP, can work in medical research to develop new drugs, evaluate existing drugs, or study drug interactions. They may also conduct clinical trials to test the safety and effectiveness of new drugs.

2. What does a medical science researcher do?

Clinical Pharmacy Specialist: Clinical pharmacy specialists work with patients to manage their medications and improve their health outcomes. They may be employed by hospitals, clinics, or pharmaceutical companies. To become a clinical pharmacy specialist, individuals typically need to have completed an MSP or PharmD degree program and obtained additional training in clinical pharmacy.

3. What does a clinical pharmacy specialist do? Where can they be employed?

---

medication /ˌmedɪˈkeɪʃn/ n.　　　　　药物;药剂;药物治疗
prescription /prɪˈskrɪpʃn/ n.　　　　　药方,处方;处方药

Hospital Pharmacy **Director**: Hospital pharmacy directors oversee the **operation** of the hospital's pharmacy department and ensure that medications are being used safely and effectively. They may also develop policies and procedures to improve patient care and reduce costs. To become a hospital pharmacy director, individuals typically need to have completed an MSP or PharmD degree program and **gained** experience in hospital pharmacy administration.

4. *What does a hospital pharmacy director do?*

Pharmaceutical Sales Representative: Pharmaceutical sales representatives promote and sell medications to healthcare professionals, such as doctors and pharmacists. They may work for pharmaceutical companies or independent **distributors**. To become a pharmaceutical sales representative, individuals typically need to have completed an MSP or PharmD degree program and obtained experience in the pharmaceutical industry.

5. *What is required to become a pharmaceutical sales representative?*

To succeed in these careers, pharmacy graduates must possess strong communication and **interpersonal** skills, as well as knowledge of medication use and side effects. They must also be able to stay **up-to-date** on the latest developments in the field of pharmacy and adhere to strict regulations **regarding** the distribution and sale of medications.

6. *What do pharmacy graduates must possess in order to succeed in the above mentioned careers?*

---

director /dɪˈrektər/ *n*.　　　　主任；主管；导演
operation /ˌɒpəˈreɪʃn/ *n*.　　　手术；运行；活动；行动
gain /geɪn/ *v*.　　　　　　　　获得；(从……中)受益；获益
distributor /dɪˈstrɪbjuːtə/ *n*.　经销商；分销商；分配者
interpersonal /ˌɪntərˈpɜːrsənl/ *adj*.　人与人之间的；人际的
up-to-date　　　　　　　　　新式的；时髦的
regarding /rɪˈɡɑːrdɪŋ/ *prep*.　关于；就……而论；至于

8.3 The Requirements for a Registered Pharmacist in China

In China, to become a registered pharmacist, individuals must meet the following requirements:

Education: Individuals must have a bachelor's degree in pharmacy or a related field from a recognized university or college. They must also pass the National Pharmacy Examination (NPEx) and obtain a license to practice as a pharmacist.

1. What is the first requirement for an individual to become a registered pharmacist?

Experience: In addition to their education, individuals must also have relevant work experience in the field of pharmacy. This can include working as a pharmacist, clinical pharmacy specialist, or other roles that require knowledge of medication use and patient care.

2. What kind of experience is needed for individuals to become a registered pharmacist?

Registration: Once individuals have met the education and experience requirements, they must apply for registration with the Chinese Pharmacist **Association**. This involves **submitting** an application, passing an examination, and meeting other requirements set by the association.

3. What is involved in a registration for a registered pharmacist?

The China Licensed Pharmacist Registration Examination (NPEx) is a national exam that assesses the knowledge and skills of pharmacists who wish to become registered in China. The exam is administered by the National Medical Products Administration (NMPA)

4. What does the NPEx assess?

---

association /əˌsəʊsɪˈeɪʃn/ *n*.　　　　协会；团体；关系；联系

submit /səbˈmɪt/ *v*.　　　　　　　　提交；递呈；顺从

and is designed to test the candidate's understanding of pharmacology, pharmacy practice, and related laws and regulations.

The NPEx consists of two parts: a written examination and a practical examination. The written examination covers topics such as drug classification, drug interactions, medication administration, and pharmacy management. The practical examination involves candidates demonstrating their ability to apply their knowledge in a real-world setting, such as dispensing medications or providing patient care.

5. What do the two parts of the NPEx cover respectively?

To pass the NPEx, candidates must score at least 75% on the written examination and meet other requirements set by NMPA. Once they have passed the exam, they are eligible to apply for registration as a licensed pharmacist in China.

It is important to note that the requirements for becoming a registered pharmacist in China may vary depending on the specific state or region in which an individual wishes to practice. Therefore, it is recommended that individuals research the specific requirements for their desired **location** before pursuing this career path.

6. What is recommended to those who wish to become a registered pharmacist in China?

8.4 The Role of Pharmacists and Their Responsibilities

Pharmacists are professional healthcare workers

1. Why are pharmacists said

location /ləʊˈkeɪʃn/ *n.*   地点;位置

who hold a degree in pharmacy. Pharmacists play a vital role in society as they are the primary healthcare providers for patients who require medication. Their responsibilities include:

Providing medication management services: Pharmacists are responsible for managing and dispensing medications to their patients. They ensure that patients receive the correct dosage, frequency, and duration of medication according to their medical condition.

Providing health education: Pharmacists are trained to provide health education to their patients about the proper use and side effects of medications. They advise patients on how to manage their medications effectively and prevent medication errors.

Monitoring patient compliance: Pharmacists are responsible for monitoring patient compliance with their prescribed medications. They review patient progress reports, **assess** medication **adherence**, and provide **counseling** when necessary.

Collaborating with other healthcare professionals: Pharmacists work closely with other healthcare professionals such as physicians, nurses, and pharmacists to **ensure** patient safety and quality care.

Advancing healthcare through research: Pharmacists are involved in drug development, clinical trials, and research projects aimed at improving the quality of care for patients.

to play a vital role in society?

2. How many responsibilities have been mentioned regarding pharmacists?

3. What health educations do pharmacists provide?

4. Why do pharmacists need to collaborate with other healthcare professionals?

---

assess /əˈses/ n .   评估;评价
adherence /ədˈhɪrəns/ n .   坚持;遵守;遵循
counseling /ˈkaʊnsəlɪŋ/ n .   咨询服务
ensure /ɪnˈʃʊə/ v .   保证;确保;担保

Overall, pharmacists play a crucial role in **maintaining** patient health and safety by providing medication management services, health education, monitoring patient compliance, collaborating with other healthcare professionals, and advancing healthcare through research.

5. How can pharmacists play a crucial role in maintaining patient health and safety?

Language Practice

I. Vocabulary Work

Complete each of the following sentences with a suitable word or expression given below.

pharmacy	pharmacist	interpersonal	assess
bachelor	certify	regarding	adherence
foundational	medication	submit	counseling
pursue	prescription	association	ensure
certification	gain	location	maintain

1. As a _____ , continuous learning and professional development are essential to advance in your career and provide the best patient care.

2. _____ to ethical guidelines and regulations is crucial for any pharmacist aiming to advance in their career and maintain a positive reputation within the industry.

3. After completing her pharmacy degree, she decided to _____ a specialization in clinical pharmacy to enhance her career prospects.

4. The pharmacy technician is working towards obtaining her _____ , which is a requirement for higher-level positions in many healthcare facilities.

5. As part of his career development plan, the pharmacy student _____ his application for a competitive internship at a leading pharmaceutical company.

6. To _____ her expertise in the field, the pharmacist regularly attends conferences and workshops to stay updated with the latest pharmaceutical

---

maintain /meɪnˈteɪn/ v.　　　　　　　　　　　　维持；维修；保养；坚称

research and regulations.

7. To build a strong career in pharmacy, it's important to have a _____ understanding of pharmacology and patient care principles.

8. During the career development process, pharmacists must _____ their own skill sets to identify areas for further education and training.

9. _____ in pharmacy informatics can open up new career paths for pharmacists interested in the intersection of technology and healthcare.

10. By participating in professional development courses, the pharmacist aims to _____ advanced knowledge in clinical pharmacology, enhancing her career prospects.

11. _____ skills training is often included in pharmacy career development programs to help professionals build rapport with patients and improve overall healthcare outcomes.

12. To advance in her career, the pharmacist is gaining expertise in behavioral _____ techniques to assist patients with chronic conditions in managing their medications effectively.

13. As part of their continuing education, pharmacists may take courses on _____ drug monitoring programs to stay updated on the latest regulations and best practices.

14. Continuing education is crucial for pharmacists to _____ they stay up-to-date with the latest medications and treatment protocols, which is essential for their career development.

15. Joining a professional pharmacy _____ can provide valuable networking opportunities and resources for career advancement in the field.

II. Word Building

Study the Prefixes, Suffixes and Roots in the following grid, and then provide the corresponding word based on the given definition.

Prefixes	Meaning	Example
cert-	"certain or sure" (肯定;确定)	certification
inter-	"between" or "among" (在……之间;在……之中)	interpersonal
en-	"to make" or "to cause" (使……)	ensure

Suffixes		
-or	"a person or thing that performs a particular action"（人或物）	distributor
-ist	"a person who specializes in a particular field or discipline"（学者；主义者）	pharmacist
Roots		
osteo	"bone"（骨）	osteopathic
found	"to lay the foundation"（奠定基础）	foundational
medic	"healing or curing"（治疗；治愈）	medication

1. to officially declare something to be true or to confirm the authenticity of something   _____

2. to make richer, especially in terms of quality or value   _____

3. a relationship in which two or more things are dependent on each other

   _____

4. a condition characterized by weakened bones that are more prone to fracture

   _____

5. the act of founding or the state of being founded; also, the base or support upon which something is built or rests   _____

6. a drug or other form of medicine used to treat or prevent illness or injury

   _____

7. a person who writes books, articles, or other literary works   _____

8. a person who studies the human mind and behavior   _____

9. relating to the treatment of illness or injury, especially by the use of drugs or other medical substances.   _____

10. a scientist who studies living organisms and their relationships with the environment   _____

III. Structure & Function

A purpose, goal or intention of the action described in the sentence can often be expressed by using a "to-do" infinitive phrase. For example：

To become a clinical pharmacy specialist, *individuals typically need to have completed an MSP or PharmD degree program and obtained additional training in clinical pharmacy.*

To become a hospital pharmacy director, individuals typically need to have completed an MSP or PharmD degree program and gained experience in hospital pharmacy administration

To succeed in these careers, pharmacy graduates must possess strong communication and interpersonal skills.

In English there are several other ways to express a purpose or goal in addition to the "to-do" infinitive phrase. For example:

She decided to pursue a degree in pharmacy in order to fulfill her dream of becoming a pharmacist.

She volunteers at a local hospital so as to improve her communication and interpersonal skills.

With the aim of becoming a doctor, she decided to major in biology.

He is currently enrolled in a pharmacy residency program for the purpose of gaining hands-on experience and improving his skills as a pharmacist.

She chose pharmacy as her profession with the intention of combining her interest in science and her desire to help others.

She is currently working as a pharmacy technician with the goal of eventually becoming a registered pharmacist.

He decided to specialize in compounding pharmacy with the objective of creating personalized medications for patients who require them.

She took courses in project management so that she could advance in her career.

Translate the following sentences, using in each an expression given in parentheses.

1. 她正在学习专业发展课程,以便跟上药学的最新趋势和进展。(in order to)

_____

_____

2. 他决定追求药剂师职业,希望通过自己的工作为人们的生活带来改变。(with the intention of)

3. 他加入了一个住院临床药师项目，以便获得该领域的深入知识和经验。（so as to）

4. 药学系的学生经常自愿在医院或社区活动中帮忙，目的是了解不同的药房环境并与其他专业人士建立联系。（for the purpose of）

5. 要成为一名临床药学专家，个人通常需要完成药学硕士或药学博士学位课程，并获得临床药学的额外培训。（to do）

IV. Audio-visual Exercise

A. Listening Comprehension

Listen to a passage，which will be spoken only once. After you hear the passage，you must choose the best answer to each question from the four choices marked A，B，C，and D.

1. Which of the following statements is NOT true of pharmacy education in China?

   A. Students are required to complete internships and practical training.

   B. Pharmacy education was focused only on TCM in the early days.

   C. Pharmacy programs include both TCM and modern pharmacy.

   D. Pharmacy education in China today is more diverse.

2. What is the basic requirement for students to become a licensed pharmacist in China?

   A. Taking the national pharmacist certification exam.

   B. Choosing to pursue a doctoral program in pharmacy.

   C. Completing a 4-year undergraduate program in pharmacy.

   D. Pursuing further education in a master's program in pharmacy.

3. One challenge facing pharmacy education in China is the need to _____ .

   A. balance theoretical teaching and practical training

   B. offer postgraduate programs that focus exclusively on TCM

   C. balance the teaching of TCM with that of Western medicine

   D. offer opportunities for students to specialize in Western medicine

4. Another challenge facing pharmacy education in China is _____ .

   A. the shortage of qualified faculty members

   B. the need to bring in international experts

   C. lack of partnerships with foreign institutions

   D. lack of enough universities to train pharmacists

5. The passage mainly deals with _____ .

   A. the role of pharmacy in China's healthcare system

   B. challenges facing pharmacy education in China

   C. demand for qualified pharmacists

   D. pharmacy education in China

B. Visual Comprehension

Watch a video clip three times and complete each of the following statements based on the video you have just watched.

1. According to the Institute of Medicine, every year, 1.5 million of the medication mistakes in the U.S. _____ .

2. The FDA is concerned about whether patients are taking their medicines _____ _____ .

3. The FDA held public meetings to ask about solutions to things like doctors prescribing the wrong medicine and pharmacists _____ _____ .

4. In spite of the FDA's efforts to prevent medication errors, the officials admit that even health care workers don't always _____ . on the bottle.

5. The FDA commissioner says their new effort goes beyond just regulating medicine and is to make sure people _____ .

V. Extended Reading

Read the following dialogue between Dr. Pharmed and students about career paths available to graduates of pharmacy, and complete each statement with a proper phrase or sentence given in the box.

Dr. Pharmed: Hello, everyone. I hope you're all doing well. Today, I want to talk to you about the various career paths available to graduates of pharmacy.

Student 1: Thank you for your time, Dr. pharmed. I'm really interested in this topic. What are some of the different jobs that pharmacy graduates can pursue?

Dr. Pharmed: There are many different career paths available to pharmacy graduates. One common option is to become a practicing pharmacist. These individuals work in drugstores or hospitals and provide patients with advice and guidance on drug usage and interactions.

Student 2: That's a great option, but I'm also interested in research. Is there a career path for pharmacy graduates in research?

Dr. Pharmed: Sure, pharmacy graduates can pursue a career in research. They can work in universities or pharmaceutical companies and focus on studying drugs and developing new medications. Additionally, they can also work on improving existing drugs and developing new applications for existing drugs.

Student 3: That's really interesting, but I want to know more about the entrepreneurial side of pharmacy. Can pharmacy graduates start their own businesses?

Dr. Pharmed: Absolutely, pharmacy graduates can start their own businesses. They can start their own pharmacies or open their own consulting firms to provide advice and guidance to other pharmacies or drug companies. Additionally, they can also start their own businesses manufacturing drugs or providing services related to pharmacy.

Student 4: That's great information, Are there any other career paths for pharmacy graduates that you would recommend?

Dr. Pharmed: Actually, there are many other career paths for pharmacy graduates. One option is to pursue a career in teaching and mentoring pharmacy students. These individuals typically work in universities and colleges teaching courses on pharmacy and counseling students on their careers. Additionally, they can also mentor students and help them develop their professional skills. Another option is to pursue a career in public health, where pharmacy graduates can work with governments and other organizations to promote healthy behaviors and policies related to pharmacy. Additionally, pharmacy graduates can also work as consultants for various organizations related to pharmacy, such as insurance companies or hospitals, to provide advice and guidance on pharmacy-related issues. Finally, pharmacy graduates can also pursue further education and become board-certified pharmacists, which allows them to specialize in specific areas of pharmacy and provide more advanced services to patients.

Student 5: Thank you so much for your time, Dr. Pharmed. This has been really helpful information for us pharmacy students who are trying to figure out our future careers.

Dr. Pharmed: You're welcome. I hope the information was helpful for you. If you have any further questions or need help figuring out your career path, feel free to come and talk to me anytime.

1. Students are really interested in _____ .
2. Practicing pharmacists provide patients with _____ .
3. Pharmacy graduates can pursue a career in research and focus on _____ .
4. Pharmacy graduates can work in universities and colleges _____ .
5. Pharmacy graduates can work as consultants for various organizations related to pharmacy to provide _____ .

> A. developing new applications for existing drugs
> B. advice and guidance on pharmacy-related issues
> C. advice and guidance on drug usage and interactions

D. various career paths available to graduates of pharmacy

E. career in government departments to promote public health

F. educating patients about appropriate use of prescription drugs

G. teaching courses on pharmacy and counseling students on their careers

VI. Topics for Discussion and Essay-writing

1. Introduce pharmacy education at multi-levels in China.

2. What are career paths available to graduate of pharmacy?

3. What are pharmacists' responsibilities as the primary healthcare providers for patients who require medication?

Appendix

Glossary

Glossary		Module
abroad /əˈbrɔːd/ *adv*.	到国外；在国外	2
absorption /əbˈsɔːrpʃ(ə)n/ *n*.	吸收；合并；同化	4
accelerate /əkˈseləreɪt/ *v*.	加速；加快	12
access /ˈækses/ *v*.	获取；获得；访问	10
accessibility /əkˌsesəˈbɪləti/ *n*.	易接近；可到达；可达性	9
accessible /əkˈsesəbl/ *adj*.	可使用的；可进入的；可理解的	9
accordance /əˈkɔːrdns/ *n*.	依照；依据；一致	11
accuracy /ˈækjərəsi/ *n*.	精确(性)；准确(性)；准确无误	9
acetaminophen /əˌsiːtəˈmɪnəfən/ *n*.	醋氨酚,对乙酰氨基酚(解热镇痛药)	3
acetylcholine /ˌæsətɪlˈkəʊliːn/ *n*.	乙酰胆碱	5
acupuncture /ˈækjʊpʌŋktʃər/ *n*.	针刺；针刺疗法	2
adapt /əˈdæpt/ *v*.	使适应/适合；改编	1
addiction /əˈdɪkʃn/ *n*.	毒瘾；着迷；嗜好	5
addictive /əˈdɪktɪv/ *adj*.	使人成瘾的；使人入迷的	10
address /əˈdres/ *v*.	解决；处理	1
adequate /ˈædɪkwət/ *adj*.	足够的；合格的；合乎需要的	10
adhere to	遵循；坚持	8
adherence /ədˈhɪrəns/ *n*.	坚持；遵守；遵循	14
administration /ədˌmɪnɪˈstreɪʃn/ *n*.	施用(药物)；实施；管理	3
adrenaline /əˈdrenəlɪn/ *n*.	肾上腺素	3
advancement /ədˈvænsmənt/ *n*.	发展；推动；提升	1
adverse /ədˈvɜːrs/ *adj*.	不利的；有害的；反面的	3
advertise /ˈædvərtaɪz/ *v*.	宣传；做广告	8
affordability /əˌfɔːdəˈbɪləti/ *n*.	支付能力；承受能力；可购性	9
affordable /əˈfɔːrdəbl/ *adj*.	价格合理的；多数人买得起的	7
AIDS (acquired immune deficiency syndrome)	获得性免疫缺乏综合征(艾滋病)	1
ailment /ˈeɪlmənt/ *n*.	疾病；病痛；微恙	1
alertness /əˈlɜːrtnəs/ *n*.	警觉；警戒；机敏	4

algorithm /ˈælgəˌrɪðəm/ n.	算法;运算法则	6
allergic /əˈlɜːrdʒɪk/ adj.	过敏的;反感的;厌恶的	4
allergy /ˈælədʒɪ/ n.	过敏反应;过敏症	3
Alzheimer's disease /ˈæltshaɪmərz dɪziːz/ n.	阿尔茨海默病	1
amoxicillin /əˌmɒksɪˈsɪlɪn/ n.	阿莫西林,羟氨苄青霉(抗生素)	4
anablioc /əˈnæbəlɪk/ adj.	合成代谢的	3
analgesics /ˌænəlˈdʒɪzɪks/ n.	止痛剂;镇痛剂	3
angiotensin /ˌændʒɪəʊˈtensən/ n.	血管紧缩素	7
antibiotics /ˌæntɪbaɪˈɒtɪks/ n.	抗生素,抗菌素	1
antidepressant /ˌæntɪdɪˈpresənt/ n.	抗抑郁剂	3
antihistamine /ˌæntɪˈhɪstəˌmɪn/ n.	抗组胺药(用于抗过敏)	3
antihyperglycemic /ˌæntɪhaɪpəglɪˈsemɪk/ adj.	抗高血糖药	8
antihypertensive /antɪhypertensɪve/ adj.	抗高血压的	7
antimicrobial /ˌæntɪmaɪˈkrəʊbɪrl/ adj.	抗菌的	7
antipsychotics /ˌæntɪpsaɪˈɒtɪks/ n.	抗精神病药	3
antipyretic /ˌæntɪpaɪˈretɪk/ adj.	退热的;退烧的	1
antitumor /ˌæntɪˈtjumər/ adj.	抗肿瘤的;抗癌的	7
antiviral /ˌæntɪˈvaɪrəl/ adj.	抗病毒的	3
appeal to /əˈpiːl tuː/	吸引;呼吁;上诉	9
approach /əˈprəʊtʃ/ n.	路径;途径;方法;方式	13
appropriate /əˈprəʊprɪət/ adj.	适当的;合适的;恰当的	7
approval /əˈpruːvl/ n.	赞成;认可;通过	6
approve /əˈpruːv/ v.	同意;批准;通过	2
assay /ˈæsˌe/ n.	检验;化验;分析	6
assess /əˈses/ n.	评估;评价	14
assessment /əˈsesmənt/ n.	看法;评估;鉴定	11
association /əˌsəʊsɪˈeɪʃn/ n.	协会;团体;关系;联系	14
atenolol /æteˈnɒlɒl/ n.	阿替洛尔,氨酰心安(β-受体阻滞剂)	3
attractive /əˈtræktɪv/ adj.	吸引人的;有魅力的;好看的	8
atypical /eˈtɪpɪkəl/ adj.	非典型的	3
authentic /ɔːˈθentɪk/ adj.	真实的;逼真的	10
authenticity /ˌɔːθenˈtɪsətɪ/ n.	真实性;可靠性;确实性	10
author /ˈɔːθər/ v./n.	创作;撰写;作者	2
authorization /ˌɔːθəraɪˈzeɪʃn/ n.	批准;授权(书)	8
automate /ˈɔːtəmeɪt/ v.	使自动化	6
avenue /ˈævənuː/ n.	途径;方法;林荫道	12
azithromycin /eɪzɪθrəˈmaɪsɪn/ n.	阿奇霉素(抗生素)	4

bachelor /ˈbætʃələr/ n.	学士；单身汉	14
bacteria /bækˈtɪrɪə/ n.	细菌	3
bacterial /bækˈtɪərɪrl/ adj.	细菌的；细菌性的	1
barrier /ˈbærɪər/ n.	障碍；壁垒；阻碍	13
be subject to	受支配；从属于	8
benzodiazepine /ˌbenzəʊdaɪˈeɪzɪpiːn/ n.	苯(并)二氮(用于制造各种镇静药)	5
beta-blocker /ˈbiːtəbˈlɒkər/ n.	[医]β-受体阻滞剂	3
bioavailability /ˌbaɪəʊrˌveɪləˈbɪlɪt/ n.	生物药效率；生物利用度	7
biochemistry /ˌbaɪəʊˈkemɪstrɪ/ n.	生物化学；生物化学过程	6
biomolecule /baɪɒmˈlɪkjuːl/ n.	生物分子	6
biopharmaceutical /baɪɒfɑːməsˈjuːtɪkl/ adj.	生物制药学	13
biotechnology /ˌbaɪəʊtekˈnɒlədʒɪ/ n.	生物技术	1
bipolar /ˌbaɪˈpəʊlər/ adj.	有两极的；双极的	3
bleeding /ˈbliːdɪŋ/ n.	出血；流血；失血	4
bond /bɒnd/ n.	纽带；联系	5
bradycardia /brædɪˈkɑːdɪə/ n.	心动过缓	7
branded /ˈbrændɪd/ adj.	有品牌的；打有烙印的	8
brand-name /ˈbrændˌneɪm/ n.	品牌名	8
breastfeeding /brestˈfidɪŋ/ v.	用母乳喂养；哺乳	5
camphor /ˈkæmfɚ/ n.	樟脑	2
candidate /ˈkændɪdeɪt/ n.	候选人；应试者；适合……的人/物	6
canon /ˈkænən/ n.	精品；真作；规范；原则	2
capsule /ˈkæpsl/ n.	胶囊；密封小容器	3
carbonyl /ˈkɑːbənɪl/ n.	碳酰基；羰基	5
cardiovascular /ˌkɑːdɪəʊˈvæskjələ(r)/ a.	心血管的	7
catalyze /ˈkætlˌaɪz/ vt.	催化；促进	5
category /ˈkætəgɔːrɪ/ n.	种类；类别	11
cellular /ˈseljələr/ adj.	细胞的；由细胞组成的；蜂窝状的	6
certificate /səˈtɪfɪkət/ n.	证明；证书	8
certification /ˌsɜːrtɪfɪˈkeɪʃn/ n.	课程结业证书；证明；鉴定	14
certify /ˈsɜːrtɪfaɪ/ v.	(出具)证明；给……颁发结业证书	14
cetirizine /sɪˈtɪrɪzɪn/ n.	西替立嗪(抗过敏药)	3
channel /ˈtʃænl/ n.	渠道；途径；门路	12
characteristic /ˌkærəktəˈrɪstɪk/ adj.	明显的；典型的；独特的	13
clozapine /kˈləʊzəpaɪn/ n.	[化]氯氮平	3
codeine /ˈkəʊdɪn/ n.	可待因(用于减轻头痛及感冒症状的药物)	3

colitis /kəˈlaɪtɪs/ n.	结肠炎	5
collaborate /kəˈlæbəreɪt/ v.	合作;协作;勾结	12
collaboration /kəˌlæbəˈreɪʃn/ n.	协作;合作	9
combat /ˈkɒmbæt/ v.	战斗;防止;减轻	9
commercialization /kəˌmɜːʃəlaɪˈzeɪʃn/ n.	商业化;商品化	6
commercialize /kəˈmɜːʃlaɪz/ v.	使商业化;以……牟利	6
comorbidity /kəmɔːˈbɪdətɪ/ n.	合并症	5
compatibility /kəmˌpætəˈbɪlətɪ/ n.	并存;相容;兼容性	11
compendium /kəmˈpendɪəm/ n.	概要;纲要	2
competition /ˌkɒmpəˈtɪʃn/ n.	竞争;比赛;竞争者;竞争产品	9
competitive /kəmˈpetətɪv/ adj.	竞争的;有竞争力的	9
competitor /kəmˈpetɪtər/ n.	竞争者;选手	9
compile /kəmˈpaɪl/ v.	汇编;编制;编纂	2
compliance /kəmˈplaɪəns/ n.	遵守;服从	11
comply with	服从;遵守	8
component /kəmˈpəʊnənt/ n.	组成部分;成分	6
compound /ˈkɒmpaʊnd/ n.	化合物;混合物	1
comprehensive /ˌkɒmprɪˈhensɪv/ adj.	综合性的;全面的	2
computational /ˌkɒmpjʊˈteɪʃənl/ adj.	计算的;计算机的	6
concern /kənˈsɜːrn/ n.	担心;令人担心的事;关心	6
conduct /kənˈdʌkt/ v.	进行;组织;实施	7
confidential /ˌkɒnfɪˈdenʃl/ adj.	机密的;保密的;悄悄的	9
confidentiality /ˌkɒnfɪˌdenʃiˈælətɪ/ n.	机密性	9
configuration /kənˌfɪɡjəˈreɪʃn/ n.	安排;布局;格局	3
conflict /ˈkɒnflɪkt/ n.	冲突;争执;战斗;矛盾	10
conform to	符合;遵照	8
confusing /kənˈfjuːzɪŋ/ adj.	难以理解的	8
conjugation /ˌkɒndʒəˈɡeɪʃn/ n.	结合	5
connectivity /ˌkɒnekˈtɪvɪtɪ/ n.	连接性;连通性	12
consent /kənˈsent/ n.	准许;同意;赞同	10
consistency /kənˈsɪstənsɪ/ n.	连贯性;一致性	9
consistent /kənˈsɪstənt/ adj.	一致的;连贯的	1
consult /kənˈsʌlt/ v.	咨询;商量;查阅	5
consumer /kənˈsuːmər/ n.	消费者;顾客	8
consumption /kənˈsʌmpʃn/ n.	消费;消耗量	8
contaminant /kənˈtæmɪnənt/ n.	污染物;致污物	9
contraindicate /ˌkɒntrəˈɪndɪkeɪt/ v.	显示(治疗)不当;禁忌(药物或疗法)	5

contraindication /ˌkɒntrəˌɪndɪˈkeɪʃn/ n.	禁忌证	5
controversial /ˌkɒntrəˈvɜːʃl/ adj.	有争议的；引发争论的	10
convert /kənˈvɜːrt/ v.	(使)转变；改造	5
coordination /kəʊˌɔːrdɪˈneɪʃ(ə)n/ n.	协调；配合；协作	4
copyright /ˈkɒpɪraɪt/ n.	版权；著作权	9
cosmetic /kɒzˈmetɪks/ n./adj.	美容品(的)；化妆品(的)	12
cost-effective /ˌkɔːst ɪˈfektɪv/ adj.	有成本效益的；划算的	12
counseling /ˈkaʊnsəlɪŋ/ n.	咨询服务	14
counterfeiting /ˈkaʊntəfɪtɪŋ/ n.	伪造	9
coursework /ˈkɔːswɜːk/ n.	(计入最终成绩的)课程作业	14
CRISPR /ˈkrɪspər/ abbr.	成簇规则间隔短回文重复序列 (Clustered Regularly Interspaced Short Palindromic Repeats)	13
criteria /kraɪˈtɪriə/ n.	标准；准则	11
cytochrome /ˈsaɪtəˌkrəʊm/ n.	细胞色素	4
database /ˈdeɪtəbeɪs/ n.	数据库	8
dataset /ˈdeɪtəset/ n.	数据集	6
dehydration /ˌdiːhaɪˈdreɪʃ(ə)n/ n.	脱水；干燥；失水	4
depression /dɪˈpreʃn/ n.	抑郁；沮丧；不景气	3
derivative /dɪˈrɪvətɪv/ n./adj.	派生物	5
descriptive /dɪˈskrɪptɪv/ adj.	描写的；叙述的	8
determine /dɪˈtɜːrmɪn/ v.	查明；测定；准确算出；决定	11
dextroamphetamine /ˌdekstrəʊæmˈfetəmɪn/ n.	右旋安非他命	5
dextromethorphan /dekstrəʊmɪˈθɔːfn/ n.	右美沙芬	5
dextrorphan /ˈdekstrɔrfn/ n.	右啡烷，右羟吗喃	5
diabetes /ˌdaɪəˈbiːtiːz/ n.	糖尿病	1
digitalization /ˌdɪdʒətələˈzeɪʃən/ n.	数字化	12
diphenhydramine /dɪfenˈhɪdrʌmən/ n.	苯海拉明，可他敏(抗过敏药)	3
director /dɪˈrektər/ n.	主任；主管；导演	14
disclose /dɪsˈkləʊz/ v.	揭露；使公开	8
disclosure /dɪsˈkləʊʒə(r)/ n.	公开；披露；揭露	10
discomfort /dɪsˈkʌmfət/ n.	不舒服；不适	7
discriminatory /dɪˈskrɪmɪnətəri/ adj.	歧视性的；区别对待；不公平的	10
dispense /dɪˈspens/ v.	分配；分发；配(药)	6
distillation /dɪstɪˈleɪʃn/ n.	蒸馏(过程)；蒸馏物	2
distinguish /dɪˈstɪŋgwɪʃ/ v.	区分；使有别于	8
distribution /ˌdɪstrɪˈbjuːʃn/ n.	分配；分布；分销	9

distributor /dɪˈstrɪbjuːtə/ n.	经销商;分销商;分配者	14
diuretics /daɪˈjʊəretɪks/ n.	利尿剂	3
diversification /daɪˌvɜːsɪfɪˈkeɪʃn/ n.	多样化;变化;多种经营	12
diversion /daɪˈvɜːrʒn/ n.	转向;转移;临时绕行路	12
docking /ˈdɒkɪŋ/ n.	对接;船停靠码头	13
domestic /dəˈmestɪk/ adj.	国内的;家用的;驯养的	11
domestically /dəˈmestɪklɪ/ adv.	在国内;在本国;家庭式	2
dopamine /ˈdəʊpəmiːn/ n.	多巴胺	4
dosage /ˈdəʊsɪdʒ/ n.	剂量;用量	3
drowsiness /ˈdraʊzɪnəs/ n.	嗜睡;睡意;昏昏欲睡	4
dynasty /ˈdaɪnəstɪ/ n.	朝代;王朝	2
e-commerce /iːˈkɒmɜːs/ n.	电子商务	12
edge /edʒ/ n.	边线;优势;影响力	9
edit /ˈedɪt/ v.	编辑;剪辑;主编	13
editing /ˈedɪtɪŋ/ n.	编辑;剪辑	13
efficacy /ˈefɪkəsɪ/ n.	功效;效力	5
Egypt /ˈiːdʒəpt/ n.	埃及	1
electrolyte /ɪˈlektrəlaɪt/ n.	电解质;电解液	4
emergence /ɪˈmɜːrdʒəns/ n.	出现;兴起	1
enhance /ɪnˈhæns/ v.	增强;提高;增加	7
enlightenment /ɪnˈlaɪtnmənt/ n.	启蒙运动;启迪;开导	1
enrollment /ɪnˈrəʊlmənt/ n.	登记;注册	13
ensure /ɪnˈʃʊə/ v.	保证;确保;担保	14
enterprise /ˈentərpraɪz/ n.	公司;企业单位	11
enzyme /ˈenzaɪm/ n.	酶	3
ester /ˈestər/ n.	酯	5
esterase /ˈestəˌreɪs/ n.	酯酶	5
ethical /ˈeθɪkl/ adj.	伦理的;道德的	6
evaluate /ɪˈvæljʊeɪt/ v.	评估;评价	6
evaluation /ɪˌvæljʊˈeɪʃn/ n.	评估;评价	6
event /ɪˈvent/ n.	事件;重大事件	2
exaggerated /ɪgˈzædʒəreɪtɪd/ adj.	夸大的;言过其实的	10
exceed /ɪkˈsiːd/ v.	(数量)超过;超越(限制、规定)	7
excretion /ɪkˈskrɪʃən/ n.	(动植物的)排泄;排泄物	5
experimentation /ɪkˌsperɪmenˈteɪʃn/ n.	实验;试验	1
expertise /ˌekspɜːrˈtiːz/ n.	专长;专门技术;专门知识	1
expired /ɪksˈpaɪəd/ adj.	过期的;失效的	9

exploit /ɪkˈsplɔɪt, ˈeksplɔɪt/ v.	利用;剥削;开采	9
explosion /ɪkˈspləʊʒn/ n.	激增;突然爆发	1
extensive /ɪkˈstensɪv/ adj.	广泛的;全面的	13
fabrication /ˌfæbrɪˈkeɪʃn/ n.	捏造;编造;制造;生产	10
facility /fəˈsɪlətɪ/ n.	设施;才能;天赋	11
falsification /ˌfɔːlsɪfɪˈkeɪʃn/ n.	伪造;弄虚作假;篡改	10
fascinating /ˈfæsɪneɪtɪŋ/ adj.	极有吸引力的;迷人的	1
fetus /ˈfiːtəs/ n.	胎;胎儿	5
feverfew /ˈfiːvərfjuː/ n.	菊科植物;白菊花	1
figure /ˈfɪgjər/ n.	人物;身影;数字	2
fine /faɪn/ n.	罚款	8
fluoxetine /fluːˈɒksətiːn/ n.	氟西汀(抗抑郁药)	4
formulate /ˈfɔːrmjʊleɪt/ v.	构想出;规划;确切地阐述	11
formulation /ˌfɔːmjəˈleʃən/ n.	(药品或化妆品的)配方;配方产品	7
foster /ˈfɑːstər/ v.	促进;鼓励;培养	9
foundational /faʊnˈdeɪʃənəl/ adj.	基本的;基础的	14
frontier /frʌnˈtɪə/ n.	前沿;新领域;边界	13
furosemide /fjʊˈrəʊsəˌmaɪd/ n.	利尿磺酸;呋胺酸;利尿灵	3
gain /geɪn/ v.	获得;(从……中)受益,获益	14
ganciclovir /gænsɪkˈləʊvə/ n.	[医]羟甲基无环鸟苷,更昔洛韦	3
gender /ˈdʒendə(r)/ n.	性别	10
generic name /dʒəˈnerɪk neɪm/ n.	通用名;总名称;属名	8
genetic /dʒəˈnetɪk/ a.	遗传的;基因的	1
genomics /dʒəˈnɒmɪks/ n.	基因组学	13
globalization /ˌgləʊbələˈzeɪʃn/ n.	全球化;全球性	12
globalize /ˈgləʊbəlaɪz/ v.	(使)全球化	12
glucuronic /gluːˈkjʊrənɪk/ adj.	葡糖醛酸	5
glucuronide /gluːˈkjʊərənaɪd/ n.	葡(萄)糖苷酸	5
glucuronyltransferase /gljuːˈkʊrənɪltrænsfrəz/ n.	葡糖醛酸基转移酶	5
grant /grænt/ v/n.	授予;允许;拨款	6
Greece /griːs/ n.	希腊	1
harmonization /ˌhɑːmənaɪˈzeɪʃn/ n.	和谐;协调;相称	11
healing /ˈhiːlɪŋ/ n.	痊愈;愈合;治愈	2
healthcare /ˈhelθkeə/ n.	卫生保健	2
heparin /ˈhepərɪn/ n.	肝(血液稀释剂)	4
herbal /ˈhɜːbl/ adj.	药草的;草本的	1
heritage /ˈherɪtɪdʒ/ n.	遗产;传统	2

high-throughput /haɪˈθruːˌpʊt/ n.	高流量	6
hinder /ˈhɪndər/ v.	阻碍;妨碍;成为阻碍	9
histamine /ˈhɪstəˌmɪn/ n.	组胺	3
HIV (Human Immunodeficiency Virus)	艾滋病病毒	1
humanely /hjuˈmeɪnlɪ/ adv.	人道地;慈悲地	10
Hydrochlorothiazide /ˌhaɪdrəˌklɒrəˈθaɪəˌzaɪd/ n.	双氢氯噻嗪,双氢克尿塞(利尿降压药)	3
hydrogen /ˈhaɪdrədʒən/ n.	氢	5
hydrolysis /haɪˈdrɒlɪsɪs/ n.	水解	5
hydrolyze /ˈhaɪdrəˌlaɪz/ v.	水解	5
hypersensitivity /ˌhaɪpəˌsensəˈtɪvətɪ/ n.	超敏反应;过敏性反应	5
hypertension /ˌhaɪpəˈtenʃn/ n.	高血压	3
hypotension /ˌhaɪpəʊˈtenʃən/ n.	低血压	7
hypothesis /haɪˈpɒθəsɪs/ n.	假设;假说;猜想;猜测	10
ibuprofen /ˌaɪbjʊˈprəʊfen/ n.	布洛芬,异丁苯丙酸(镇痛消炎药)	3
ibuprofenone /ˈaɪbjʊˈprɒfən/ n.	与布洛芬相关的化学衍生物	5
identification /aɪˌdentɪfɪˈkeɪʃn/ n.	识别;鉴定;确认	6
idiosyncratic /ˌɪdɪəsɪʔˈkrætɪk/ adj.	特异应性的;特异体质的;乖僻的	7
illegal /ɪˈliːɡl/ adj.	不合法的	9
imbalance /ɪmˈbæləns/ n.	失衡;失调;不安定	4
immunosuppression /ˌɪmjʊnəʊsəˈpreʃn/ n.	免疫抑制	7
impair /ɪmˈpeə/ v.	损害;削弱;妨碍	4
implement /ˈɪmplɪment, ˈɪmplɪmənt/ v.	实施;执行;使生效	9
implication /ˌɪmplɪˈkeɪʃn/ n.	可能的影响;含意;牵连	10
importation /ˌɪmpɔːˈteʃən/ n.	进口;输入;进口货	11
impurity /ɪmˈpjʊrətɪ/ n.	掺杂;不纯;混杂物;污点	9
in vitro	在生物体外进行的;用试管进行的	10
incur /ɪnˈkɜːr/ vt.	招致;引起;遭受	9
independent /ˌɪndɪˈpendənt/ adj.	不相关的;不受影响的;独立的	10
indication /ˌɪndɪˈkeɪʃn/ n.	适应证;表明;标示	7
ineffective /ˌɪnɪˈfektɪv/ adj.	无效果的;无效率的	8
infection /ɪnˈfekʃn/ n.	传染;感染;传染病	1
influencer /ˈɪnflʊənsər/ n.	有影响的人(或事物)	12
influential /ˌɪnflʊˈenʃl/ adj.	有影响力的;有权势的	2
informed /ɪnˈfɔːmd/ adj.	了解情况的;有见识的;有根据的	10
ingredient /ɪnˈɡriːdɪənt/ n.	组成部分;(烹调的)原料	8
inhibit /ɪnˈhɪbɪt/	抑制;禁止;阻止	3

inhibitor /ɪnˈhɪbɪtə/ n.	抑制剂;抑制者	3
inhumane /ˌɪnhjuːˈmeɪn/ adj.	残忍的;不人道的	10
injection /ɪnˈdʒekʃn/ n.	注射;打针;投入	3
innovation /ˌɪnəˈveɪʃn/ n.	创新;新观念;新发明	1
innovative /ˈɪnəveɪtɪv/ adj.	创新的;革新的;新颖的	12
insight /ˈɪnsaɪt/ n.	洞察力;领悟;了解	12
inspection /ɪnˈspekʃn/ n.	检查;检验;视察	11
institution /ˌɪnstɪˈtuːʃn/ n.	机构;社会收容机构;习俗	11
integrity /ɪnˈtegrətɪ/ n.	正直,诚实;完整	10
intellectual /ˌɪntəˈlektʃʊəl/ adj.	智力的;有才智的;需用智力的	8
interact /ˌɪntərˈækt/ v.	相互作用;交流;互动	13
interaction /ˌɪntərˈækʃ(ə)n/ n.	相互作用;互动;沟通	4
interchangeable /ˌɪntərˈtʃeɪndʒəbl/ adj.	可交换的;可交替的	8
interferon-alpha /ˌɪntəˈfɪrɒnˈælfə/ n.	[医]α-干扰素	3
internal /ɪnˈtɜːrnl/ adj.	内部的;体内的;国内的	2
interpersonal /ˌɪntərˈpɜːrsənl/ adj.	人与人之间的;人际的	14
interpolation /ɪnˌtɜːpəˈleɪʃn/ n.	插值;内插;补充部分	10
intervention /ˌɪntərˈvenʃn/ n.	介入;干预;干涉	12
iterative /ˈɪtəˌreɪtɪv/ adj.	重复的;反复的;迭代的	13
jurisdiction /ˌdʒʊrɪsˈdɪkʃn/ n.	司法权;管辖权	8
keep track of	跟踪;记录	7
kidney /ˈkɪdnɪ/ n.	肾;肾脏	5
labeling /ˈleɪblɪ/ n.	标贴;标志	8
laborious /ləˈbɔːrɪəs/ adj.	耗时费力的;辛苦的;艰难的	13
lactation /lækˈteʃən/ n.	哺乳期	5
lawsuit /ˈlɔːsuːt/ n.	诉讼;诉讼案件	8
legal /ˈliːgl/ adj.	合法的	8
legitimacy /lɪˈdʒɪtɪməsɪ/ n.	合法(性);合理(性);正当(性)	10
liability /ˌlaɪəˈbɪlətɪ/ n.	责任;倾向;债务	8
liable /ˈlaɪəbl/ adj.	有责任的;有义务的	8
license /ˈlaɪsns/ n.	许可证;特许	8
lifesaving /ˈlaɪfˌseɪvɪ/ adj.	救命的;救生的	1
literature /ˈlɪtrətʃər/ n.	著述;文献;文学;文学作品	6
lithium /ˈlɪθɪəm/ n.	锂	4
location /ləʊˈkeɪʃn/ n.	地点;位置	14
logo /ˈləʊgəʊ/ n.	标识;标志;徽标	8
loratadine /lreɪteɪˈdaɪn/ n.	氯雷他定(抗组胺药)	3

macromolecule /ˌmækrəˈmɒləˌkjʊl/ *n.*	高分子;巨大分子	6
maintain /meɪnˈteɪn/ *v.*	维持;维修;保养;坚称	14
makeup /ˈmeɪˌkʌp/ *n.*	组成成分;构成;构造	13
malaria /məˈleɪrɪə/ *n.*	疟疾	1
malicious /məˈlɪʃəs/ *adj.*	恶意的;有敌意的;蓄意的	9
manipulate /məˈnɪpjʊleɪt/ *v.*	操作;处理;控制	13
manufacturer /ˌmænjʊˈfæktʃərər/ *n.*	制造商;制造厂	8
manufacturing /ˌmænjəˈfæktʃərɪŋ/ *n.*	制造;加工;工业	2
mediate /ˈmiːdɪeɪt/ *v.*	影响;调节;调停	4
medication /ˌmedɪˈkeɪʃn/ *n.*	药物;药剂;药物治疗	14
medicinal /mɪˈdɪsənəl/ *adj.*	药用的;治疗的	1
memorable /ˈmemərəbl/ *adj.*	难忘的;值得纪念的;显著的	8
metabolite /meˈtæbəˌlaɪt/ *n.*	代谢物	5
metabolize /məˈtæbəlaɪz/ *v.*	使新陈代谢	3
metformin /metˈfɔːmɪn/ *n.*	二甲双胍(抗糖尿病药、降血糖药)	8
metoprolol /metɒpˈrɒlɒl/ *n.*	美托洛尔(β-受体阻滞剂)	3
microfluidics /maɪkrəʊfluˈɪdɪks/ *n.*	微流体	12
minimize /ˈmɪnɪmaɪz/ *v.*	使减至最低程度;使保持最低程度	7
misleading /mɪsˈliːdɪŋ/ *adj.*	误导性的;骗人的;引入歧途的	8
modality /məʊˈdælətɪ/ *n.*	模式;方式	1
modeling /ˈmɒdlɪŋ/ *n.*	建模;造型(术)	10
molecular /məˈlekjələr/ *adj.*	分子的;与分子有关的	13
molecule /ˈmɒlɪkjuːl/ *n.*	分子;微小颗粒	5
monitoring /ˈmɒnɪtərɪŋ/ *n.*	监控;监视;监督	6
monoamine /ˌmɒnəʊˈmin/ *n.*	单胺;一元胺	3
monopoly /məˈnɒpəlɪ/ *n.*	垄断;专卖;垄断者;专利品	9
morphine /ˈmɔːfin/ *n.*	吗啡	5
multidisciplinary /ˌmʌltɪdɪsəˈplɪnərɪ/ *adj.*	包括各种学科的;多学科的;多部门的	11
musk /mʌsk/ *n.*	麝香	2
myelosuppression /maɪˈləʊsʌpreʃn/ *n.*	骨髓抑制	7
nandrolone /ˈnændrəˌləʊn/ *n.*	诺龙(可提高运动成绩的违禁药品)	3
nanotechnology /ˌnænəʊtekˈnɒlədʒɪ/ *n.*	纳米技术	13
naproxenone /nəˈprɒksən/ *n.*	与萘普列克松相关的化合物	5
neurodegenerative /ˌnjʊrəʊdɪˈdʒenərətɪv/ *adj.*	神经组织退化的	6
neurotransmitter /ˈnʊrəʊtrænzmɪtər/ *n.*	神经传递素	3
neutral /ˈnuːtrəl/ *adj.*	中性的;中立的;暗淡的	4

pharmacopoeia /ˌfɑːməkəˈpɪə/ n.	药典	2
pharmacy /ˈfɑːrməsɪ/ n.	药学;药剂学;药房;制药业	14
phenothiazine /ˌfinəʊˈθaɪəˌzin/ n.	吩噻嗪(用作杀虫剂或药物制造)	3
physician /fɪˈzɪʃn/ n.	医生;内科医生	1
physiology /ˌfɪzɪˈɒlədʒɪ/ n.	生理学;生理(功能)	2
piracy /ˈpaɪrəsɪ/ n.	盗版行为;非法复制;海上抢劫	9
plasma /ˈplæzmə/ n.	血浆;原生质;细胞质	1
policymaker /ˈpɒlɪsɪˌmeɪkə/ n.	政策制订者;决策人	9
postdoctoral /ˌpəʊstˈdɒktərəl/ adj.	博士后的	14
post-marketing	上市后	8
postwar /ˈpəʊstˈwɔː/ a.	战后的	1
potency /ˈpəʊtnsɪ/ n.	效力;药力;药效	6
precaution /prɪˈkɔːʃn/ n.	预防措施;防备	7
precision /prɪˈsɪʒn/ n.	精确;精密	12
preclinical /prɪˈklɪnɪkəl/ adj.	临床应用前的;潜伏期的	6
predict /prɪˈdɪkt/ v.	预言;预测;预告	13
prediction /prɪˈdɪkʃn/ n.	预测;预报;预言	13
pregnancy /ˈpregnənsɪ/ n.	怀孕;妊娠;丰富	5
premium /ˈpriːmɪəm/ adj.	优质的;高昂的	9
prescribe /prɪˈskraɪb/ v.	开处方;给医嘱;规定	1
prescription /prɪˈskrɪpʃn/ n.	药方;处方;处方药	14
primarily /praɪˈmerɪlɪ/ adv.	首要地;主要地	1
primary /ˈpraɪmərɪ/ adj.	首要的;最早的;初级的	10
proactive /ˌprəʊˈæktɪv/ adj.	积极的;主动的;主动出击的	12
procedure /prəˈsiːdʒər/ n.	程序;步骤	8
profile /ˈprəʊfaɪl/ n.	侧面;半面;轮廓	6
promising /ˈprɒmɪsɪŋ/ adj.	很有前途的;前景很好的	13
promote /prəˈməʊt/ v.	促进;促销;晋升	9
promptly /ˈprɒmptlɪ/ adv.	立即;迅速地;及时	7
pronounce /prəˈnaʊns/ v.	发……的音;宣称;宣布	8
property /ˈprɒpərtɪ/ n.	特性;属性;财产	1
propranolol /prəʊˈprænəˌlɒl/ n.	普兰洛尔,心得安(β-受体阻滞剂)	3
proprietary /prəˈpraɪətərɪ/ adj.	专有的;专利的	8
prosecute /ˈprɒsɪkjuːt/ v.	控告;起诉;继续从事;担任控方律师	9
protein /ˈprəʊtiːn/ n.	蛋白质	6
provincial /prəˈvɪnʃəl/ adj.	省的,州的;领地的;地方的	11
provision /prəˈvɪʒn/ n.	提供;供给	10

psychoactive /ˌsaɪkəʊˈæktɪv/ *adj.*	对精神起作用的;影响精神行为的	5
purchase /ˈpɜːtʃəs/ *v.*	购买;采购	12
purity /ˈpjʊərətɪ/ *n.*	纯度;纯洁;纯净	9
purposeful /ˈpɜːpəsfl/ *adj.*	有明确目的的;故意的;果断的	10
pursue /pərˈsuː/ *v.*	寻求;追求;继续	14
pursuit /pərˈsuːt/ *n.*	追求;寻求	1
quinine /ˈkwaɪˌnaɪn/ *n.*	奎宁,金鸡纳霜	1
radiotherapy /ˌreɪdɪəʊˈθerəpɪ/ *n.*	放疗	1
rash /ræʃ/ *n.*	疹子;皮疹	7
real-time	即时处理的;实时的	13
receptor /rɪˈseptər/ *n.*	感受器;受体	3
recognition /ˌrekəgˈnɪʃn/ *n.*	认识;识别;认出	2
refill /riˈfɪl/ *n.*	重新配药	7
reflect /rɪˈflekt/ *v.*	反映;表现;反射	2
reform /rɪˈfɔːrm/ *n.*	改革;改善	9
regarding /rɪˈgɑːrdɪŋ/ *prep.*	关于;就……而论;至于	14
regimen /ˈredʒɪmən/ *n.*	养生法;养生之道;生活规则	13
register /ˈredʒɪstər/ *v.*	给……注册;登记	8
registration /ˌredʒɪˈstreɪʃn/ *n.*	注册;登记;挂号	8
registry /ˈredʒɪstrɪ/ *n.*	登记处	8
regulatory /ˈregjələtɔrɪ/ *adj.*	监管的;具有监管权的;调整的	6
relevant /ˈreləvənt/ *adj.*	相关的;相应的;适当的	12
reliable /rɪˈlaɪəbl/ *adj.*	可靠的;可信赖的;真实可信的	10
relieve /rɪˈliːv/ *v.*	缓和;缓解;减轻	3
remedy /ˈremədɪ/ *n.*	药品;治疗方法	1
Renaissance /ˈrenəsɑːns/ *n.*	文艺复兴	1
renal /ˈrɪnəl/ *adj.*	肾脏的;肾的	7
replication /ˌreplɪˈkeɪʃn/ *n.*	复制;折叠	3
reproducibility /rɪˌprədjuːsəˈbɪlɪtɪ/ *n.*	再现性;复现性;可重现性	10
reproducible /ˌriprəˈdjuːsəbl/ *adj.*	可复现的;可再生的	10
reputation /ˌrepjʊˈteɪʃn/ *n.*	名誉;名声	8
requirement /rɪˈkwaɪərmənt/ *n.*	要求;必要条件	8
resistance /rɪˈzɪstəns/ *n.*	抗药性;抵抗力;阻力	4
resource /ˈriːsɔːrs/ *n.*	资源;物力;财力	12
respiratory /ˈrespərətɔːrɪ/ *adj.*	呼吸的	7
retention /rɪˈtenʃn/ *n.*	保持;保留	3
reuptake /riˈʌpteɪk/ *n.*	重新吸收;重新摄取	3

review /rɪˈvjuː/ n.	评审;检查;评论	11
Reye's syndrome	雷依氏综合征	5
ribavirin /ˈraɪbəˌvaɪrɪn/ n.	三唑核苷,病毒唑(抗病毒药)	3
rigorously /ˈrɪɡərəslɪ/ adv.	严密地;严厉地;残酷地	9
robotic /rəʊˈbɒtɪk/ adj.	机器人的;自动的	6
salicylic /ˌsæləˈsɪlɪk/ adj.	水杨酸的	5
scale /skeɪl/ n.	规模;等级;标度	12
schizophrenia /ˌskɪtsəˈfriːnɪə/ n.	精神分裂症	3
screening /ˈskriːnɪŋ/ n.	筛选;筛查	6
sedative /ˈsedətɪv/ adj.	镇静的;有镇静作用的;有催眠作用的	4
seizure /ˈsiːʒər/ n.	癫痫;疾病突然发作;没收	4
selective /sɪˈlektɪv/ adj.	选择性的;有选择的	3
selectivity /sɪˌlekˈtɪvɪtɪ/ n.	选择性;专一性	6
sensitive /ˈsensətɪv/ adj.	敏感的;过敏的;灵敏的	8
serotonin /ˌserəˈtəʊnɪn/ n.	血清素	3
sexual /ˈsekʃʊəl/ adj.	性的;与性别有关的;有关性行为的	10
significant /sɪɡˈnɪfɪkənt/ adj.	重要的;显著的;意味深长的	2
simulation /ˌsɪmjʊˈleɪʃn/ n.	模仿;模拟;仿真品	13
simultaneously /ˌsaɪməlˈteɪnɪəslɪ/ adv.	同时地;同步地;一齐	12
slogan /ˈsləʊɡən/ n.	短语;标语;口号	8
slurred /slɜːrd/ adj.	含糊不清的;含含糊糊的;含混的	4
solely /ˈsəʊllɪ/ adv.	唯一地;仅仅	9
span /spæn/ v.	横跨;跨越;包括	1
specification /ˌspesɪfɪˈkeɪʃn/ n.	规格;详述;说明书	11
spironolactone /spaɪˈrɒnəˌlækˌtəʊn/ n.	螺旋内酯甾酮(利尿药)	3
split /splɪt/ v./n.	分裂;分开;裂缝	5
sponsoring /ˈspɒnsərɪŋ/ n.	赞助;资助	8
stability /stəˈbɪlətɪ/ n.	稳定(性);稳固;坚定	11
stakeholder /ˈsteɪkhəʊldə(r)/ n.	股东;利益相关者	9
standardize /ˈstændərdaɪz/ v.	使标准化;使合乎标准	1
stanozolol /stæˈnɒlɒl/ n.	吡唑甲基睾丸素(雄激素性合成类固醇)	3
status /ˈsteɪtəs/ n.	地位;状态;情形	13
steroid /steˈrɔɪd/ n.	类固醇;甾类化合物	3
stifle /ˈstaɪfl/ v.	遏制;扼杀;镇压	9
strategy /ˈstrætədʒɪ/ n.	战略;策略;部署	12

streamline /ˈstriːmlaɪn/ v.	使(过程等)精简;效率更高	13
strengthen /ˈstreŋθn/ v.	巩固;加强;增强	9
streptomycin /ˌstreptəˈmaɪsɪn/ n.	链霉素	3
stroke /strəʊk/ n.	中风;脑卒中	4
submit /səbˈmɪt/ v.	提交;递呈;顺从	14
suboptimal /ˈsʌbˈɒptɪməl/ adj.	未达最佳标准的;不最适宜的;不最满意的	9
substandard /sʌbˈstændəːd/ adj.	不够标准的;在标准以下的;低等级标准	9
substantial /səbˈstænʃl/ adj.	大量的;重大的;结实的	9
sulfate /ˈsʌlˌfeɪt/ n.	硫酸盐	5
sulfotransferase /sʌlfətrænsfˈreɪz/ n.	转磺酶;磺基转移酶	5
supervision /ˌsjuːpəˈvɪʒn/ n.	监督;管理	10
supplier /səˈplaɪər/ n.	供应商;供应国;供应者	11
surgical /ˈsɜːdʒɪkl/ adj.	外科的;外科手术的	1
surveillance /sɜːrˈveɪləns/ n.	监督;管制	8
switch /swɪtʃ/ v.	转换;改变;转变	13
synthesis /ˈsɪnθəsɪs/ n.	合成;综合	1
synthesize /ˈsɪnθəsaɪz/ v.	合成;人工合成	1
synthetic /sɪnˈθetɪk/ adj.	合成的;人造的	6
tailor /ˈteɪlər/ v.	量身打造;按需定制	1
tap into	利用;开发	12
target /ˈtɑːrɡɪt/ n.	靶子;目标;对象	6
terminate /ˈtɜːrmɪneɪt/ v.	(使)终止;(使)结束	13
terminology /ˌtɜːrmɪˈnɒlədʒɪ/ n.	术语;专门名词;术语学	8
testosterone /teˈstɒstərəʊn/ n.	睾酮;睾丸素(男性荷尔蒙的一种)	3
tetracycline /ˌtetrəˈsaɪklɪn/ n.	四环素	3
The Compendium of Materia Medica	《本草纲目》	2
The Yellow Emperor's Inner Canon	《黄帝内经》	2
therapeutic /ˌθerəˈpjuːtɪk/ adj.	治疗(学)的;疗法的	1
time-consuming /ˈtaɪm kənsuːmɪŋ/ adj.	耗时的;费时的	13
tirelessly /ˈtaɪələslɪ/ adv.	不知疲倦地;坚韧地	1
tissue /ˈtɪʃuː/ n.	组织;薄纸;面巾纸	13
tolerance /ˈtɒlərəns/ n.	忍耐(力);忍受(力);耐药性	13
toxic /ˈtɒksɪk/ adj.	有毒的;毒性的;中毒的	4
toxicity /tɒkˈsɪsətɪ/ n.	毒性;毒力	6
track down	追查出;追寻;查获	9

trademark /ˈtreɪdmɑːrk/ n.	(注册)商标	8
trait /treɪt/ n.	特点;特征;特性	12
transform /trænsˈfɔːrm/ v.	转换;改变;改造	13
transfusion /trænsˈfjuːʒn/ n.	输血	1
transmission /trænzˈmɪʃ(ə)n/ n.	传输;传递;传送	4
transparency /trænsˈpærənsɪ/ n.	透明;透明度;透明性	9
tremor /ˈtremər/ n.	颤抖;战栗;哆嗦	4
trial /ˈtraɪəl/ n.	试验;试用;审讯	6
tricyclic /traɪˈsɪklɪk/ adj.	三环的	3
truthful /ˈtruːθfl/ adj.	真实的;如实的;诚实的	10
tuberculosis /tjʊˌbɜːkjəˈləʊsɪs/ n.	肺结核;结核病	1
ulcerative /ˈʌlsərətɪv/ adj.	溃疡(性)的	5
undergo /ˌʌndərˈɡəʊ/ v.	经历;忍受	8
unethical /ʌnˈeθɪkl/ adj.	不道德的	10
unique /juˈniːk/ adj.	独有的;特有的	7
up-to-date	新式的;时髦的	14
validate /ˈvælɪdeɪt/ v.	证实;确认;使有法律效力	6
validation /ˌvælɪˈdeɪʃn/ n.	确证;确认;证明……有价值	13
version /ˈvɜːrʒn/ n.	版本;变体	9
vessel /ˈvesl/ n.	血管;容器;船舰	3
viral /ˈvaɪrəl/ adj.	病毒的;病毒引起的	3
vital /ˈvaɪtl/ adj.	必要的;至关重要的;充满活力的	2
vulnerable /ˈvʌlnərəbl/ adj.	易受伤害的;脆弱的	10
warfarin /ˈwɔːrfərɪn/ n.	华法林(血液稀释剂)	4
welfare /ˈwelfeə(r)/ n.	幸福;安全与健康;福利	10
withdrawal /wɪðˈdrɔːəl/ n.	撤回;退出	5
witness /ˈwɪtnəs/ v.	见证;目击	1

Teaching Module Contents

（教学单元概览）

Chapter	Module		Word Building	Structure	Audio-visual Exercise	Extended Reading
I Overall Introduction to Pharmacy	1 1.1	Overview of the Development of Pharmaceutical Science	anti-, post-, -ical, -osis, -ology, pharmac, bio, syn	Attributive clauses 定语从句	Spot Dictation *The history of pharmaceutical science* Visual Comprehension *Cancer drug breakthrough*	The development of pharmaceutical science
	2 1.2	Overview of the Pharmaceutical Development in China	ab-, manu-, -ant, -age, -ium, signify physio herit	The passive structure 被动语态	Spot Dictation *The development of pharmaceutical science in China* Visual Comprehension *The First cancer drug targeting a tumor solely based on its DNA*	The history of pharmaceutical development in China

续 表

Chapter	Module	Word Building	Structure	Audio-visual Exercise	Extended Reading
	3 2.1 Drug Classification	intra-, bi-, -olol, -ics, -oid, -ological, alg, venous	To + infinitive phrase 动词不定式短语	Spot Dictation *Why it is important to follow drug instructions* Visual Comprehension *Miracle drug: Aspirin*	The classification of pharmaceuticals
II Basic Knowledge of Drugs	4 2.2 Drug Dosage and Dosage Forms 2.3 Drug Actions	cyto-, de-, -ness, -arin, -illin, -etine, chromo, electr(o)	Gerund phrases 动名词短语	Spot Dictation *Drug actions and effects on the body* Visual Comprehension *Dangerous Drug Overdose*	Drug interactions and contraindications
	5 2.4 Drug Interactions 2.5 Drug Contraindications 2.6 Drug Metabolism	hyper-, oxi-, -itis, ulcerate, contra, morbid, hydro, psycho	Expressions of contrast 对比表达法	Sentence Dictation Visual Comprehension *Michael Jackson Death: Lethal Drug Dosage*	Drug metabolism

续　表

Chapter	Module	Word Building	Structure	Audio-visual Exercise	Extended Reading
III Research and Development of Drugs	6 3.1 The Basic Process of Drug Research and Development 3.2 Key Technologies and Tools in Drug Development	peri-, robo-, -ation, -al, bio, merce, val, cell	The present participle 现在分词短语	Sentence Dictation Visual Comprehension *What You Need to Know about COVID-19 Vaccine Development*	The basic process of drug research and development
IV Clinical Application of Drugs	7 4.1 Issues Involved in Drug Clinical Application 4.2 Drug Indications 4.3 Drug Adverse Reactions 4.4 Precautions for Medication	re-, mini-, -ory, -ly, path(o), micro, respire, cardio	Modal verbs 情态动词	Sentence Dictation Visual Comprehension *Hidden Risk of Medication*	Drug adverse reactions
V Legal and Ethical Issues of Drugs	8 5.1 Drug Naming 5.2 Drug Registration Procedures 5.3 Drug Advertisements	non-, mis-, in-, -able, -ive, sens, intellect, surveil	The past participle 过去分词语	Sentence Dictation Visual Comprehension *Are Drug Ads Misleading?*	Drug registration procedures
	9 5.4 Drug Pricing	sub-, im-, -ability, -ible,	Expressions of reason	Sentence Dictation	Drug quality issues

续 表

Chapter	Module	Word Building	Structure	Audio-visual Exercise	Extended Reading
	5.5 Quality of Drugs 5.6 Intellectual Property Rights of Drugs	-cy, mal, access, contam	原因表达法	Visual Comprehension *How Effective Are Generic Drugs?*	
	10 5.7 Animal Testing 5.8 Research Integrity 5.9 Marketing Ethics	dis-, un-, hypo-, -ful, -sion, -ure, legit, sent	Conjunction+ ellipsis 连接词＋省略句结构	Listening comprehension *Research integrity in drug R & D* Visual Comprehension *Doctor Faked Research*	Intellectual property rights
VI Safety Regulation of Drugs	11 6.1 Implementation of Inter-national Pharmaceutical Standards 6.2 Implementation of China's Pharmaceutical Stand-ards 6.3 Safety Assessment and Quality Control of Drugs	out-, com-, over-, -ment, -tion, accord, spect, import	Nominaliza-tion 名词化结构	Listening comprehension *International pharmaceutical standards* Visual Comprehension *Drug Bust Pfizer Fined for Fraud*	The safety assessment and quality control of drugs

续 表

续 表

Chapter	Module	Word Building	Structure	Audio-visual Exercise	Extended Reading
	8.3 The Requirements for a Registered Pharmacist in China 8.4 The Role of Pharmacists and Their Responsibilities	osteo, found, medic	目的/目标表达法	Visual Comprehension *Preventing Medication Errors*	

图书在版编目 (CIP) 数据

药学概要 : 英文/陈社胜总主编 ; 关庆等主编.
上海 : 复旦大学出版社, 2024. 9. ——(复旦博学).
ISBN 978-7-309-17534-9

Ⅰ. R9

中国国家版本馆 CIP 数据核字第 202435PZ30 号

药学概要
陈社胜　总主编
关　庆　等　主编
责任编辑/贺　琦

复旦大学出版社有限公司出版发行
上海市国权路 579 号　邮编 : 200433
网址 : fupnet@ fudanpress. com　http://www. fudanpress. com
门市零售 : 86-21-65102580　团体订购 : 86-21-65104505
出版部电话 : 86-21-65642845
浙江临安曙光印务有限公司

开本 787 毫米×1092 毫米　1/16　印张 13.75　字数 246 千字
2024 年 9 月第 1 版第 1 次印刷

ISBN 978-7-309-17534-9/R · 2107
定价 : 52.00 元